HEALTH AND HUMAN DEVELOPMENT SERIES

CONCEPTUALIZING BEHAVIOUR IN HEALTH AND SOCIAL RESEARCH: A PRACTICAL GUIDE TO DATA ANALYSIS

Health and Human Development Series
Joav Merrick, Series Editor

Adolescent Behavior Research: International Perspectives
Joav Merrick and Hatim A. Omar
2007. ISBN: 1-60021-649-8

Complementary Medicine Systems: Comparison and Integration
Karl W. Kratky
2008. ISBN: 978-1-60456-475-4

Pain in Children and Youth
Patricia Schofield and Joav Merrick
2008. ISBN: 978-1-60456-951-3

Behavioral Pediatrics, 3rd Edition
Donald E. Greydanus, Dilip R. Patel, Helen D. Pratt and Joseph L. Calles, Jr.
2009. ISBN: 978-1-60692-702-1

Behavioral Pediatrics, 3rd Edition
Donald E. Greydanus, Dilip R. Patel, Helen D. Pratt and Joseph L. Calles, Jr.
2009. ISBN: 978-1-60876-630-7 (Online Book)

**Health and Happiness from Meaningful Work:
Research in Quality of Working Life**
Søren Ventegodt and Joav Merrick
2009. ISBN: 978-1-60692-820-2

Obesity and Adolescence: A Public Health Concern
Hatim A. Omar, Donald E. Greydanus, Dilip R. Patel and Joav Merrick
2009. ISBN: 978-1-60456-821-9

Poverty and Children: A Public Health Concern
Alexis Lieberman and Joav Merrick
2009. ISBN: 978-1-60741-140-6

**Living on the Edge: The Mythical, Spiritual, and Philosophical
Roots of Social Marginality**
Joseph Goodbread
2009. ISBN: 978-1-60741-162-8

Challenges in Adolescent Health: An Australian Perspective
David Bennett, Susan Towns, Elizabeth Elliott and Joav Merrick (Editors)
2009. ISBN: 978-1-60741-616-6

Challenges in Adolescent Health: An Australian Perspective
David Bennett, Susan Towns, Elizabeth Elliott and Joav Merrick (Editors)
2009. ISBN: 978-1-61668-240-8 (Online Book)

Alcohol-Related Cognitive Disorders: Research and Clinical Perspectives
Leo Sher, Isack Kandel and Joav Merrick
2009. ISBN: 978-1-60741-730-9

Alcohol-Related Cognitive Disorders: Research and Clinical Perspectives
Leo Sher, Isack Kandel and Joav Merrick
2009. ISBN: 978-1-60876-623-9 (Online Book)

Advances in Environmental Health Effects of Toxigenic Mold and Mycotoxins- Volume 1
Ebere Cyril Anyanwu
2010. ISBN: 978-1-60741-953-2

Children and Pain
Patricia Schofield and Joav Merrick (Editors)
2009. ISBN: 978-1-60876-020-6

Child Rural Health: International Aspects
Erica Bell and Joav Merrick (Editors)
2010. ISBN: 978-1-60876-357-3

Conceptualizing Behavior in Health and Social Research: A Practical Guide to Data Analysis
Said Shahtahmasebi and Damon Berridge
2010. ISBN: 978-1-60876-383-2

Chance Action and Therapy. The Playful Way of Changing
Uri Wernik
2010. ISBN: 978-1-60876-393-1

Adolescence and Chronic Illness. A Public Health Concern
Hatim Omar, Donald E. Greydanus, Dilip R. Patel and Joav Merrick (Editors)
2010. ISBN: 978-1-60876-628-4

Adolescence and Sports
Dilip R. Patel, Donald E. Greydanus, Hatim Omar and Joav Merrick (Editors)
2010. ISBN: 978-1-60876

International Aspects of Child Abuse and Neglect
Howard Dubowitz and Joav Merrick
2010. ISBN: 978-1-60876-703-8

Positive Youth Development: Evaluation and Future Directions in a Chinese Context
Daniel T.L. Shek, Hing Keung Ma and Joav Merrick (Editors)
2010. ISBN: 978-1-60876-830-1

Positive Youth Development: Evaluation and Future Directions in a Chinese Context
Daniel T.L. Shek, Hing Keung Ma and Joav Merrick (Editors)
2010. ISBN: 978-1-61668-376-4 (Online Book)

Pediatric and Adolescent Sexuality and Gynecology: Principles for the Primary Care Clinician
Hatim A. Omar, Donald E. Greydanus, Artemis K. Tsitsika, Dilip R. Patel and Joav Merrick (Editors)
2010. ISBN: 978-1-60876-735-9

Understanding Eating Disorders: Integrating Culture, Psychology and Biology
Yael Latzer, Joav Merrick and Daniel Stein (Editors)
2010. ISBN: 978-1-61668-261-3.

Advanced Cancer Pain and Quality of Life
Edward Chow and Joav Merrick (Editors)
2010. ISBN: 978-1-61668-207-1

Positive Youth Development: Implementation of a Youth Program in a Chinese Context
Daniel T.L Shek, Hing Keung Ma and Joav Merrick (Editors)
2010. ISBN: 978-1-61668-230-9

HEALTH AND HUMAN DEVELOPMENT SERIES

CONCEPTUALIZING BEHAVIOUR IN HEALTH AND SOCIAL RESEARCH: A PRACTICAL GUIDE TO DATA ANALYSIS

SAID SHAHTAHMASEBI
AND
DAMON BERRIDGE

Nova Science Publishers, Inc.
New York

Copyright © 2010 by Nova Science Publishers, Inc.

All rights reserved. No part of this book may be reproduced, stored in a retrieval system or transmitted in any form or by any means: electronic, electrostatic, magnetic, tape, mechanical photocopying, recording or otherwise without the written permission of the Publisher.

For permission to use material from this book please contact us:
Telephone 631-231-7269; Fax 631-231-8175
Web Site: http://www.novapublishers.com

NOTICE TO THE READER

The Publisher has taken reasonable care in the preparation of this book, but makes no expressed or implied warranty of any kind and assumes no responsibility for any errors or omissions. No liability is assumed for incidental or consequential damages in connection with or arising out of information contained in this book. The Publisher shall not be liable for any special, **consequential, or exemplary damages resulting, in whole or in part, from the readers' use of, or** reliance upon, this material.

Independent verification should be sought for any data, advice or recommendations contained in this book. In addition, no responsibility is assumed by the publisher for any injury and/or damage to persons or property arising from any methods, products, instructions, ideas or otherwise contained in this publication.

This publication is designed to provide accurate and authoritative information with regard to the subject matter covered herein. It is sold with the clear understanding that the Publisher is not engaged in rendering legal or any other professional services. If legal or any other expert assistance is required, the services of a competent person should be sought. FROM A DECLARATION OF PARTICIPANTS JOINTLY ADOPTED BY A COMMITTEE OF THE AMERICAN BAR ASSOCIATION AND A COMMITTEE OF PUBLISHERS.

LIBRARY OF CONGRESS CATALOGING-IN-PUBLICATION DATA

Shahtahmasebi, Said.
  Conceptualizing behavior : a practical guide to data analysis / Said Shahtahmasebi and Damon Berridge.
      p. cm.
  Includes bibliographical references and index.
  ISBN 978-1-60876-383-2 (hbk.)
 1. Psychology--Statistical methods. 2. Social sciences--Statistical methods. 3. Psychology--Research--Methodology. 4. Social sciences--Research--Methodology. I. Berridge, Damon. II. Title.
  BF39.S4325 2009
  150.72'7--dc22
                                                                                        2009036326

Published by Nova Science Publishers, Inc. ✦ *New York*

CONTENTS

Preface xi

Acknowledgment xii

Chapter 1 Introduction 1
   1.1. Introduction 1
   1.2. Some Important Analytical Issues 5
      1.2.1. Explanatory Variables 5
      1.2.2. Multicollinearity 5
      1.2.3. Error-in-Variables or Measurement Error 6
      1.2.4. Residual Heterogeneity/Omitted Variables 6
      1.2.5. Temporal Dependence and Past Behaviour 7
      1.2.6. Non-Stationarity 7
      1.2.7. Data: Cross-Sectional and Longitudinal 8
      1.2.8. Causality 10
   1.3. Framework for Inference: 10
   Statistical Modelling 10
   1.4. Attrition/Drop out 12
   1.5. Data Sources Used in this Book 12

Chapter 2 Statistical Modelling of Survival in Old Age 13
   2.1. Introduction 13
   2.2. Background 14
   2.3. Data Description and Exploratory Analyses 14
   2.4. Statistical Modelling of Binary Survival in Old Age 18
      2.4.1. Variable Selection 21
      2.4.2. Interpretation 22
      2.4.3. Summary 23
   2.5. Statistical Modelling of Multinomial Survival in Old Age 25
      2.5.1. Statistical Approach and Assumptions 26
      2.5.2. Model Specification 26
      2.5.3. Variable Selection 28
      2.5.4. Interpretation 29
      2.5.5. Summary 33

	2.6. Statistical Modelling of Duration Dependence: Survival in Old Age	34
	2.6.1. Statistical Modelling of Survival Times	35
	2.6.2. Problem 1: Missing Durations	35
	2.6.3. Problem 2: A Substantive Issue	36
	2.6.4. Operationalisation of the Model with Missing Durations	36
	2.6.5. Variable Selection Process	37
	2.6.6. Interpretation	39
	2.7. Summary	40
	2.8. Conclusions	41
Chapter 3	**Statistical Modelling of Morale in Old Age**	**43**
	3.1. Introduction	43
	3.2. Morale in Old Age: Background	44
	3.3. Data	45
	3.4. Analytical Issues	46
	3.4.1. Continuous Response Variable	46
	3.4.2. Multicollinearity	47
	3.4.3. Past Behaviour	47
	3.4.4. Omitted Variables	48
	3.4.5. Subjectivity	48
	3.5. Strategies for Analysis	49
	3.6. Cross-Sectional Analysis of Baseline Data	49
	3.6.1. Variable Selection Process	50
	3.6.2. Testing for Subjectivity	50
	3.6.3. Unrestricted Model	51
	3.6.4. Interpretation of Table 3.3	51
	3.7. Pooled Cross-Sectional Analysis	52
	3.7.1. Interpretation of Table 3.5	54
	3.8. Longitudinal Modelling of Morale in Old Age	56
	3.8.1. Methods of Controlling for Time-Constant Residual Heterogeneity	58
	3.8.2. Longitudinal Analysis of Morale in Old Age	60
	3.8.3. Controlling for Time-Variant Omitted Variables: Instrumental Variables Revisited	69
	3.8.4. Concluding Remarks	72
Chapter 4	**SABRE**	**77**
	4.1. Introduction	77
	4.2. Statistical Models in SABRE	78
	4.2.1. Event History Models	79
	4.2.2. Stayers, Nonsusceptibles and Endpoints	79
	4.2.3. State Dependence	80
	4.2.4. Linear Model with Fixed Effects	80
	4.3. Installing and Using SABRE	81
	4.4. Example of a Sample Run	81

	4.5. SABRE Applications for this Book	83
	4.5.1. Model Fitting in SABRE: Commands to Fit	
	a Binary Logistic Model	84
	4.5.2. Model Fitting in SABRE:	89
	Commands to Fit an Ordinal Logistic Model	89
	4.5.3. Model Fitting in SABRE:	91
	Commands to Fit Bivariate Binary Logistic Model	91
	4.6. Using SABRE with Commercial Packages	95
Chapter 5	**Examples of SABRE Application**	**97**
	5.1. Introduction	97
	5.2. Example 1: Univariate Binary Response	97
	5.2.1. Teenage Smoking	97
	5.3. Example 2: Multinomial (Ordinal) Response	106
	5.3.1. Teenage Alcohol Drinking	106
	5.4. Example 3: Bivariate Binary Response	116
	5.4.1. Linguistic Innovation in London	116
Chapter 6	**Conclusions**	**121**
References	**Appendix I – List of Explanatory Variables**	**141**
	A. List of Variables Used in Survival Analysis Sections (Chapter 2)	141
	B. List of Variables Used in the Analysis of Morale	
	in Old Age (Chapter 3)	142
	C. Further Details of Explanatory Variables listed	
	in sections a and b	142
	D. Network Type	143
	Appendix II – Binary Response Model	145
	I. Probability of Survival (Success)	145
	II. Calculating Non-Survival	145
	Appendix III – Multinomial Response Model	146
	Appendix IV – Duration Dependence Model	149
	Appendix V – A Sufficient Statistic for a Binary Response	151
	Appendix VI – Marginal Likelihood	151
	Method for a Continuous Response	151
	Appendix VII – Marginal Likelihood Method	
	for a Binary Response	153
	Appendix VIII – Errors in Variables and Instrumental Variables	155
	Appendix IX – Controlling for Time-Variant Omitted Variables	157
	Appendix X – SABRE Commands	161
BIOSKETCH		**171**
Index		**173**

PREFACE

The emphasis in this book is not on the mathematics of statistics nor is it on technical aspects or statistical assumptions. These are discussed in numerous other books and relevant journals. The emphasis in this book is to *unpack* statistical thinking. This is done through anticipation and expectation of difficult issues to be addressed in real life examples and by outlining ways of dealing with them as they arise. Thus, it is intended to illustrate the application of statistical concepts in order to gain insight into the subject under investigation by appropriate development of the cognitive aspects of research. Without due consideration to substantive issues when analysing data, even the application of appropriate statistical techniques may lead to mis-interpretation of results and misleading conclusions. This is a very serious consequence in particular in an environment where evidence-based practice has been encouraged.

The idea of this book was borne out of frustration when dealing with policy makers, or senior academic colleagues involved with researching evidence to advise politicians/policy makers. This activity in itself is an interesting field that requires a holistic treatment, i.e. to be studied as a human behaviour. The main issue is the disparity between 'evidence' and the process of policy formation. This misalignment has led to the development of a culture in which policy development tends to use evidence selectively (e.g. see (1)). In other words, supportive evidence is sought after a policy has been formed. Regardless of any political consequences, this approach ignores the feedback effects on social and individual parameters. Over recent years the vocabulary of political language has been expanded to include 'evidence-based' decision-making, although there tends to be confusion over what exactly constitutes 'evidence'. **But, when politicians cite 'evidence-based' it is often directed at other** professionals! Even so, when evidence is found, the policy formation process fails to assess critically its value and its contribution in informing the process. This feedback effect may well have its roots in education which trains potential policy analysts for the established culture, i.e. numbers, proportions and schematic as opposed to critical thinking. Similarly, phrases such as 'dynamics' and 'social processes' or 'dynamics of social processes' are being used more frequently. It is essential to account for the fact that *dynamism* may be due, at least in part, to human activities, e.g. social governance through socio-economical and educational policies. For example, within the disability literature and policy maker circles, there is a raging debate about the effect of a child disability on family hardship, income and health, and vice versa. Often this dynamic is translated into the proportion of change in each outcome group on which inference about the population is based. These types of conclusions will lead to a 'scattergun' approach to policy making and further complexities due to feedback effects.

In general, this book is an attempt to encourage a discussion of the main substantive issues and how they may have an impact on the statistical methodology and the interpretation of results. Furthermore, we hope to have provided some motivation to promote the practice and adoption of analytical methods that allow for statistical control.

ACKNOWLEDGMENT

We would like to thank our Commissioning Editor, Professor Joav Merrick, and editorial team at Nova Science Publishing for their patience and encouragement with this book.

We would like to thank Dr Eivind Torgersen, Senior Research Associate, Department of Linguistics and English Language, Lancaster University, for his kind permission to use the 'Linguistic innovation in London' data in Chapter 5.

Chapter 1

INTRODUCTION

1.1. INTRODUCTION

This book is not about statistics made simple, basic statistics, statistics for dummies or anything to do with the mathematics of statistics. There are many books on the mathematical aspects of statistics, statistical computing and inference. The interested reader is advised to search their library. Quite simply, this handbook is about the issues that are raised and discussed in the behavioural sciences but which are very rarely addressed in the design of the study or allowed for within the framework for analysis. As an example, consider the number of times you have come across the phrase 'dynamics of a process'. As another example, consider the fashionable phrase 'evidence-based decision-making' in particular within the health industry. Reflect upon what is meant by these phrases when they were so frequently used by professionals and academics alike, and how these ideas have been translated into action and practice. Comedians appear to be profound observers of the dynamics of human behaviour which may make them good at anlysing and commenting on such issues as evidence-based policy making, for example: '… **since most accidents** occur at home, the Royal Society for the Prevention of Accidents advise you to move!' (the Two Ronnies, BBC).

Over the recent decades, there has been much emphasis on evidence-based practice to justify a new policy or changes in existing policy. A question arises: what constitutes evidence? In terms of human behaviour, evidence is the means by which we choose to justify an action or a decision. Frequently, action may be taken ahead of evidence gathering (e.g. see [1]). Under this elective model, supportive evidence is sought selectively subsequent to policy implementation. Certainly, under alternative models, hypothesis testing and randomized clinical trials (RCTs) do not constitute evidence in isolation to justify a change to existing policy or in introduction of a new policy. Although RCTs play a role in the pharmaceutical industry, they have very limited use when investigating issues related to human behaviour. Whether an elective model or other types of model are applied, perhaps, it is our uncritical **use of the 'evidence' that is the weakness** and ultimately the cause of us taking a flawed decision.

Human behaviour, like deterministic physical models, will respond to an input, but human reaction unlike the output of deterministic models is not always measurable or quantifiable exactly. For example, measuring health status through a survey questionnaire **may lead to the informant's health being described** as e.g. excellent, good, allright, poor, very poor. Such measurements or description of a variable will be influenced by the informant's own general well being at the time of the interview, as well as his/her personal and social traits. It is plausible that informants may assess their health status by giving consideration to other factors e.g. personal expectation and the feel good factor. For example, elderly people may describe their poor health as being allright (for their age) [2]. The complexities arise when we attempt to infer cause and effect from the health status variable to another variable such as morale, employment status, smoking, longevity or loneliness. Cross-sectionally, the health effect may appear to be statistically significant. However, longitudinally, changes in health status may not lead to commensurate changes in morale i.e. over time, **individuals'** state of health change but their morale levels may remain unchanged. Figures 1.1 and 1.2 may illustrate the point more clearly. In a large study of the relationship between presence of child disability and other family related outcomes, the outcome profiles of each family can be ploted against time. The profiles for two such families, labeled X.1 and X.2, are plotted in Figures 1.1 and 1.2. For instance, Figure 1.1 shows that there was no child disability in family X.1 in 2001, this changed in 2002 and a child disability remained for the rest of the project window. However, this change does not appear to coincide with a change in family hardship, income poverty or health. Although there appears to be an improvement in the latter in 2005, three years after the incidence of a child disability. On the other hand, the moderate hardship of family X.2 shown in Figure 1.2 appears to coincide with the occurrence of child disability in the family. A change in health status **from 'good' to 'fair'** is reported in 2004 and there is no reported change in income hardship. Several issues arise: (a) it is unsafe to make statements about a causal relationship **if the family's past history is unknown; (b) there may** be those families who persistently remain is one state e.g. severe hardship or no hardship; (c) there may be those families who move between states e.g. from good health to poor health and back to good health; (d) some families may take a long time to react to a change in circumstances; (e) the period of adjustment will vary between families and by type of disability.

On the other hand, analytical methodology is just as important as appropriate translation of substantive issues into study and statistical issues. The application of cross-sectional methods to longitudinal data leads to assumption violation and misleading results. Often it is this mis-specification in cross-sectional models that inflates the importance of relationships between explanatory variables and an outcome variable.

Even when the analytical methodology has been appropriately chosen we must always bear in mind that we are dealing with human behaviour. In other words, there are other human traits, such as frailty, personality and the good feel factor, that cannot be measured and thus are omitted from surveys. Such unobserved variables will have an impact on the outcome through an unobserved association with observed explanatory variables. As an extreme but simple example consider the outcome of national lottery: probability models calculate the chance of an individual winning the lottery to be small (almost zero) but on average there is a jackpot winner on a regular basis!

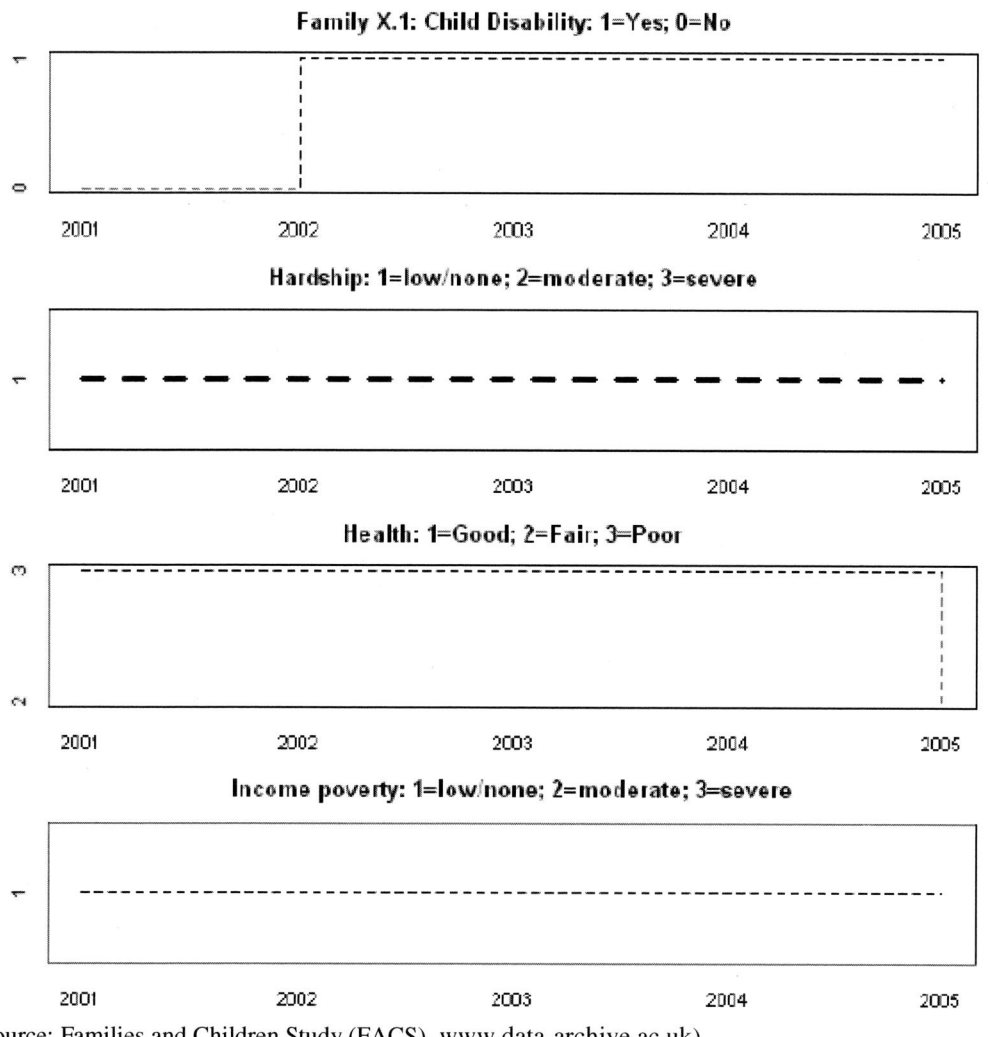

Source: Families and Children Study (FACS), www.data-archive.ac.uk).

Figure 1.1. Profiles of child disability and other outcomes.

A theoretical and philosophical discussion of human behaviour is not presented in this book. The key message is that, when studying human behaviour, in particular with a view to informing policy development, temporal dependencies must be taken into account. The following anecdotes quoted in the media serves to demonstrate the consequences of adopting an uncritical approach and by not accounting for temporal dependencies. On the MMR controversy in the UK, the BBC reported (http://news.bbc.co.uk/1/hi/health/1808826.stm) that some studies linked the MMR vaccine to autism whilst others offered evidence to the contrary. The BBC also reported that, on the one hand, 'Alcohol makes your brain grow: Drinking alcohol boosts the growth of new nerve cells in the brain, research suggests.' (http://news.bbc.co.uk/go/em/-/1/hi/health/4496727.stm), and on the other hand 'Alcohol link to bowel cancer risk: A daily pint of beer or a large glass of wine raises the risk of bowel cancer by about 10%, research suggests.' (http://news.bbc.co.uk/go/em/-/1/hi/health/6921998.stm). In New Zealand, the media took delight in reporting and quoting research from the US, on how alcohol can improve memory! Given the effects that alcohol has on living cells and on human health, such reported outcomes are counter intuitive at best, yet the emphasis is often on the word 'research' thus resulting in an uncritical and unquestioning acceptance of research outcomes. Indeed, for every claim from one group of scientists there would have been a counter claim. In suicide research, Beautrais [3-5] claimed that depression and mental illness were the cause of suicide and Khan et al [6] claimed that antidepressants did not reduce suicide rates and may increase the risk of suicide, while Hall et al [7] claimed that antidepressants reduced suicide rates. These studies have failed to address methodological issues related to design, data collection and analysis thus resulting in misleading conclusions [8, 9]. We believe that such research and reporting has considerably attenuated the credence and prestige that research once had in the mind of the public.

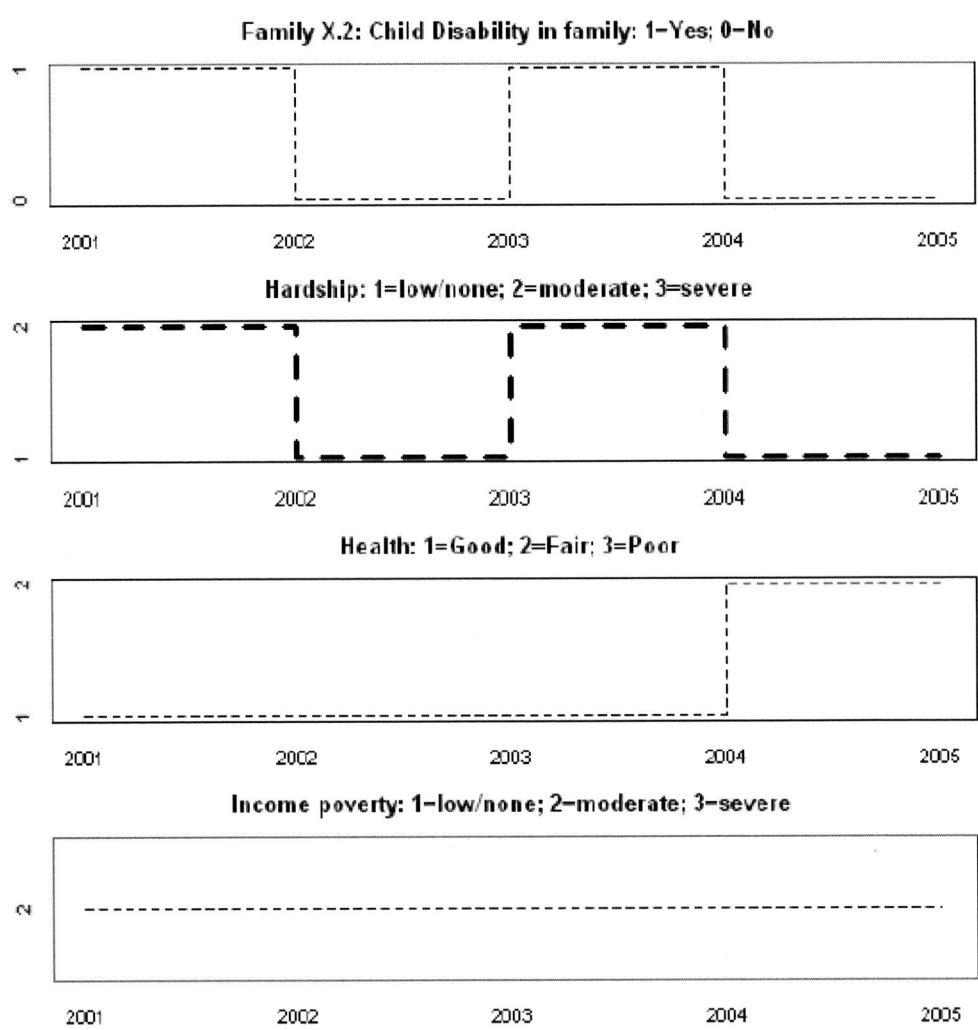

Source: Families and Children Study (FACS), www.data-archive.ac.uk).

Figure 1.2. Profiles of child disability and other outcomes.

In recent decades, there have been methodological developments, mainly in the field of econometrics (e.g. see [10, 11]) and in longitudinal analysis (modelling) which, to some extent, have overcome problems with assumption violations and other related issues (discussed in the subsequent section). These methodologies have been further developed in the social sciences with applications to social survey data (e.g. see [12-14]). In particular, the most important development has been to allow simultaneous control for measured and omitted variables (e.g see [15-17]).

The rest of this chapter is concerned with a discussion of the main issues that arise when dealing with data from observational studies.

1.2. SOME IMPORTANT ANALYTICAL ISSUES

1.2.1. Explanatory Variables

Explanatory variables are observed/recorded characteristics such as age, sex and state of health on each inidividual. In relation to the process outcome under study, some of these variables will be endogenous and some will be exogenous. Exogenous variables are those that affect the process externally. That is, the values of such variables cannot change as a result of the process e.g. in relation to morale in old age, age of the elderly people and social class based on their last job before retiring are exogenous variables. Endogenous variables are those that affect the process internally and there may be some feed-back. For example when modelling health care, 'health' can be an endogenous variable. The task of identifying endogenous and exogenous variables depends on the outcome under investigation. This issue can be problematic when 'feed-back' is present in the process and it may lead to overestimation or underestimation of the effects of explanatory variables [16, 18].

1.2.2. Multicollinearity

The inter-relationships between explanatory variables are often referred to as multicollinearity. This issue is illustrated with a simple example from Wallace and Silver [19]. Consider the Venn diagrams in Figure 1.3, where circle Y represents the total variation in Y (response variable), and the circles X_1 and X_2 correspond to the total variation in X_1 and in X_2 respectively. Figure 1.3(a) represents a situation in which X_1 and X_2 are uncorrelated; there is no overlap in the variation of the Xs. The blacked-out areas represent the total variation in Y that is explained by the X's. The 'net effect' of X_1 and X_2 on Y is the same as their 'gross effect' (blacked-out areas). Figure 1.3(b) shows a situation in which there is variation common to all three variables. In this example, the net effect of X_1 on Y includes the effect of X_2. To determine the 'net effect' of X_1 on Y the effect from X_2 must be removed (this is the grey area). Now suppose that the circle X_2 is completely encompassed within the circle X_1. Having taken into account the effect of X_1 on Y, X_2 is redundant i.e. cannot explain any further variation in Y. This latter situation is often referred to as perfect multicollinearity.

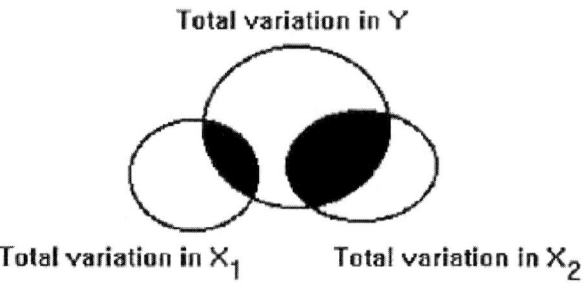

(a) X_1 and X_2 uncorrelated; net effects equal to gross effects

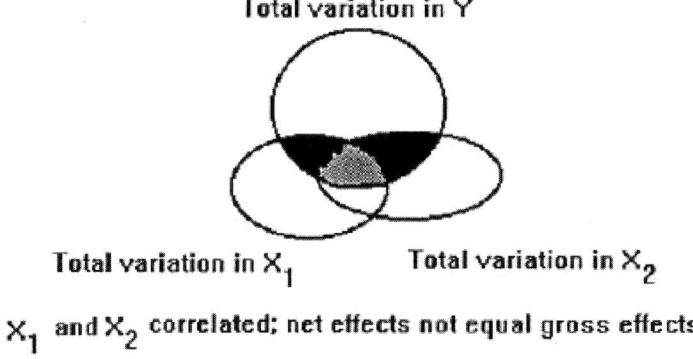

(b) X_1 and X_2 correlated; net effects not equal gross effects

Figure 1.3. Venn diagram representation of multicollinearity.

1.2.3. Error-in-Variables or Measurement Error

Measurement error is a more common and frequent problem with social survey data. The problem occurs when measuring certain characteristics which are measurable but cannot be quantified precisely. For example, age and sex are measurable and quantifiable, while state of health is often self-reported as perceived by the respondent. Such measures as perceptions, self reported variables and attitudes may not reflect the 'true' value of the variables being measured. For instance, elderly people tend to under report poor health [20]. Similarly, men are reported to be less willing to admit to loneliness. This problem with observational data tends to lead to an underestimation or overestimation of the effects of explanatory variables (e.g. see [19]).

1.2.4. Residual Heterogeneity/Omitted Variables

Residual heterogeneity is defined to be the effect of variables omitted from the study because either they are unmeasurable (e.g. frailty or the feel good factor) or they cannot be quantified within a social survey study (e.g. biological factors). In social studies of human behaviour, the effects of residual heterogeneity can be complex. For example, it is possible that when modelling a statistical association between a response variable and an explanatory variable (e.g. between morale and state of health), the response, or both variables, may be dependent upon an unobserved variable (e.g. frailty). Therefore, to avoid erroneous results, the analysis must include an explicit representation of residual heterogeneity [14-16], see Figure 1.4.

1.2.5. Temporal Dependence and Past Behaviour

Often, in studies of social behaviour, the interest lies not only in the individual's current outcome, but also upon whether there is a relationship with past behavioural patterns and whether they will influence future patterns, see Figure 1.4. In such studies, the interest centres on change over time i.e. after adjusting for change in observed characteristics, the current value of the outcome may be significantly related to its previous value(s). Suppose the outcome is loneliness and we find that various factors, including age and entry into residential care, are related to loneliness. Now suppose that a retrospective study of individuals' life histories reveals a high prevalence of loneliness prior to entry into care. Perhaps lonely elderly people are more likely to go into residential homes. That is, residential homes may not be the cause of loneliness but being lonely in the first place is the reason for entry into residential homes.

Results from a USA study [21] suggested that the farther away a person lived from the respondent, the more likely they were to be emotionally close! This was counter to results from other work which tended to suggest frequency of interaction as a predictor of emotional closeness: living far apart would mean less frequent interaction and less emotional closeness. The author argued that the *duration* of friendship could hold the key to explaining the counter intuitive results.

In general, a process may depend on the previous state of its own outcome. This type of temporal dependence is often referred to as state dependence. It is sometimes the case that the outcome process is dependent on duration in the current state. This is referred to as duration dependence. This issue can be the source of complex problems but, if omitted from the model, may lead to overestimation of the effects of explanatory variables.

1.2.6. Non-Stationarity

Non-stationarity is defined as the temporal variation in the exogenous variables in the outcome process. For example, changes in the state of health of elderly individuals through effective health care policy (or through changes in health care policy) may influence the probability of survival. Therefore, feedback becomes a more complex issue. The response variable is influenced by its own past levels which have been subject to an outside influence through observed explanatory variable(s). The modelling of feedback processes can be simplified if the processes are stationary [22]. However, most social processes are not stationary. The above issues may be visualised graphically in Figure 1.4.

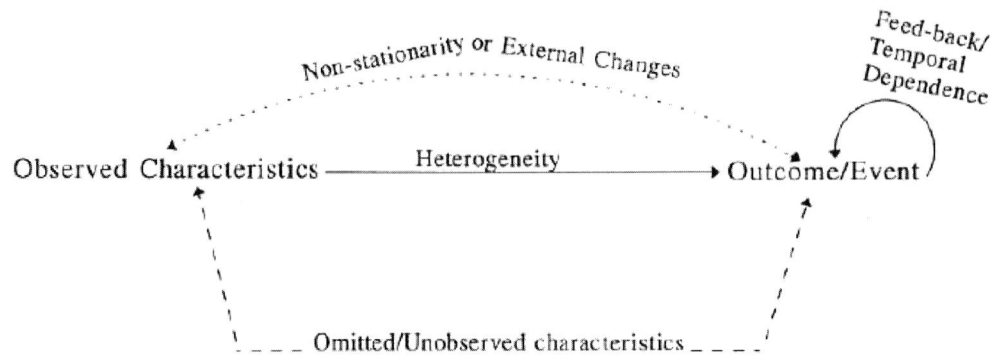

Figure 1.4. Graphical illustration of sources of variation in observational studies.

1.2.7. Data: Cross-Sectional and Longitudinal

Observations made on individuals at one particular point in time are often referred to as *cross-sectional* data, for example see Figure 1.5. Cross-sectional data are useful in providing information on the characteristics of a population (e.g. demographic, socio-economic), and to ilicit knowledge about an outcome process. They can also be informative about the process of change; for example, the variables **'number of years widowed'**, **'previous occupation'**, **'home tenure a year earlier'** serve as descriptors of an elderly **person's life history**. As shown in Figure 1.5 this type of data, whilst being partially informative about the past, essentially remains cross-sectional. There is only one link from the explanatory variables to the current state of the response variable. In contrast, longitudinal data (Figure 1.6) follow the same individuals over time, thus providing repeated observations on the response and explanatory variables. The main differences between cross-sectional data (Figure 1.5) and longitudinal data (Figure 1.6) can be summarized as:

a   cross-sectional data include information on variation between individuals, while longitudinal data include information on *variation within* as well as variation between individuals,

b   with cross-sectional data, the prevalence of an outcome can be investigated. With longitudinal data, in addition to examining the prevalence of an outcome, we can also explore changes in prevalence. Longitudinal data may also be used to identify those individuals who always or almost always remain in the same state in contrast to those who always or almost always move between states (known as movers).

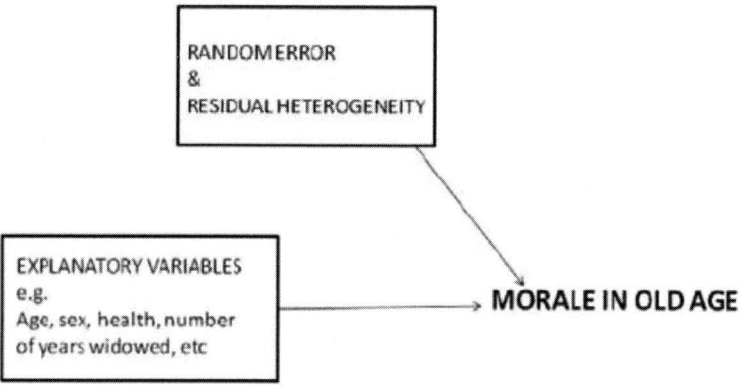

Figure 1.5. Graphical representation of cross-sectional data.

Specifically, Figures 1.5 and 1.6 demonstrate the limitation of cross-sectional data for investigating social processes. With the longitudinal scheme (Figure 1.6) the individual observed at time t_1 is observed again at t_2 (Figure 1.6). In effect, individuals at t_1 are their own controls at t_2 thereby informing us of change within individuals and enabling us to distinguish residual heterogeneity from the random error. Such a sampling design allows us to address a number of issues, which were discussed earlier and are shown in Figure 1.6. Having repeated observations on the same individuals assists us in establishing the role of explanatory variables while controlling for feed-back or past behaviour, non-stationarity and residual heterogeneity.

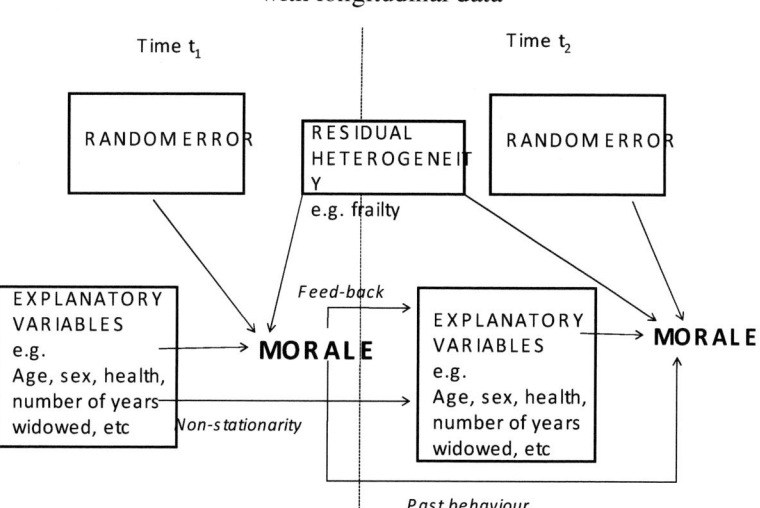

Figure 1.6. Graphical representation of issues that can be studied with longitudinal data.

1.2.8. Causality

Direction of causality is also an important feature of a dynamic process. A consequence of ignoring, or reaching erroneous conclusions about, the direction of causality is to add more confusion and complexities to the dynamics of a process. These additional complexities are introduced to a process through feed-back by policies which are based on erroneous conclusions on causality. There are several examples of this problem [14]. Perhaps the most well-known and well-publicised is the ambiguous cross-sectional link between ill-health and unemployment: 'it has not in general been possible to distinguish between ill-health leading to unemployment and unemployment causing ill-health' (a quote from Peter West, in [16]). Another example in the study of human behaviour which may be noted from Figures 1.4 and 1.5 is the relationship between the state of health and levels of morale in old age: does ill-health lead to a lower morale, or could low morale cause ill-health? Methods have been proposed for establishing direction of causality, but, as will be seen in Chapter 3, a pragmatic approach has been adopted to tackle this problem in this book.

1.3. FRAMEWORK FOR INFERENCE: STATISTICAL MODELLING

The emphasis in this book is to present a comprehensive framework for inference [23, 24] to distinguish systematic effects in the data from random variation which tends to obscure any pattern. 'Statistical modelling' is a comprehensive structured framework for making inference from data. The statistical modelling approach may be summarised as follows (e.g. see [25]):

a Model formulation - this step involves the consideration of a well thought out sampling scheme and the type of data in hand. It is guided by substantive theory. In summary, for generalized linear modeling [25]:

    i. express the mean or 'expected' value of the response variable as a function of explanatory variables and a vector of parameters or regression coefficients;
    ii. define a probability distribution for an observed value of the response variable about its expected value (which may require further unknown parameters).

b Model fitting - the resulting parsimonious model from (a) is then fitted using likelihood theory. The general principle of statistical inference states that all the sample information is contained in the likelihood function. Moreover, 'best supported' values of parameters are those which maximise the likelihood function.

c Model criticism - having 'best' estimates for the parameters, the current model can then be tested to see how well it explains the data. For example, goodness of fit measures, likelihood ratio statistics and examination of residuals may be used.

Introduction

If, as a consequence of (a) and (b), the current model is proves satisfactory then proceed with the interpretation of the model using substantive theory else repeat steps (a)-(c).

Many conventional statistical techniques tend to use hypothesis testing. Within the statistical modelling framework, hypothesis testing has a role to play in selecting the most parsimonious model and, in this context, hypothesis testing is a logical part of the comprehensive analysis. This is in contrast to conventional statistical analysis in which hypothesis testing tends to be seen as an independent inferential statement often of meagre substantive value.

For the *non-statistician,* grappling with *statistical modelling* is more of a challenge because of its explicit emphasis on *probability modelling*.

In this book, we attempt to address some of the above issues which are summarised in Figure 1.7 (also see Heckman and Borjas [26]), through exercising statistical *control* using data from real life examples. Chapter 2 deals with an example involving survival in old age progressively. Chapter 2 presents complex models starting with analyses of a simple binary outcome before proceeding to models for multinomial and continuous outcomes. In Chapter 3, the focus will move to modelling of repeated observations (analysis of longitudinal data) with a continuous outcome. The theme of Chapter 3 is morale in old age. Statistical modelling illustrated in Chapter 3 id defined within both cross-sectional and longitudinal study frameworks. In both Chapters 2 and 3, we highlight and discuss difficult issues arising from survey type studies and demonstrate ways of dealing with them. Chapter 4 provides a full discussion of SABRE (Software for the Analysis of Binary Recurrent Events). SABRE's most recent features and examples of SABRE applications are provided in Chapter 5. Chapter 6 summarises the main issues raised in this book using further examples.

Fig. 1.7 Sources of variation

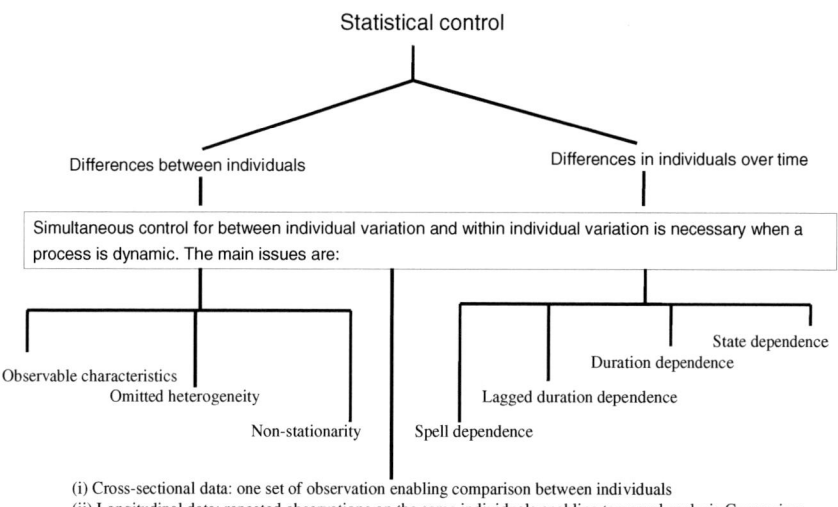

Figure 1.7. Sources of variation.

1.4. ATTRITION/DROP OUT

There will inevitably be missing data due to sample attrition or drop out of informants in longitudinal studies. Attrition or drop out will lead to bias if missing data are in some way informative about the response variable under study, and therefore, must be allowed for within the analytical framework. There are methods of dealing with this problem e.g. see [27]. Throughout this book, we have adopted a pragmatic approach to deal with this problem as and when encountered.

1.5. DATA SOURCES USED IN THIS BOOK

The data for Chapters 2 and 3 came from the North Wales Elderly Project (NWEP) (see [2, 28]). In NWEP, a sample of elderly people living in North Wales (UK) in 1979 were surveyed using an extensive questionnaire. All the subjects were traced after 4 and 8 years i.e. in 1983 and 1987 respectively, and their status was recorded as to whether they were still in the community, were in care, had moved out of the area or had deceased (see Table 1.1). Due to the funding structure only the sample of old elderly (those who were 75 years old in 1979) was surveyed in 1983. Many of the explanatory variables that had been reported in the literature were then extracted from the database.

1979	1983	1987
534 respondents (aged 65+) were interviewed	First follow up of the sample: 108 old elderly re-interviewed; 117 deceased; 17 in residential care.	Second follow up of the sample: all survivors re-interviewed; 107 deceased since 1983; 29 in residential care.

Table 1.1. The structure of the NWEP longitudinal data.

The data for the teenage smoking and teenage drinking pattern examples in Sections 5.2 and 5.3 came from the Yorkshire (UK) Health Related Behaviour Questionnaire [29, 30], see Section 5.2.1.2.

The data for the bivariate binary example in Section 5.4 came from the project *Linguistic innovators: the English of adolescents in London* [31]. This project studied whether ethnicity is a significant determinant of variation in the spoken English of young working-class people in London. In this study design, the speech of a group of speakers was recorded and played back to a sample of listeners. After listening, the listeners were required to make a guess on the ethnicity of the speaker (white, black, Asian or other) and the locality (Hackney or Havering) they came from, see Section 5.4.1.2.

Chapter 2

STATISTICAL MODELLING OF SURVIVAL IN OLD AGE

2.1. INTRODUCTION

In Chapter 1, we highlighted some of the main issues relevant to studies of human behaviour that researchers must grapple with. The importance of dealing with such analytical issues appropriately was highlighted. An understanding of the issues discussed in Chapter 1 provides the researcher with a lever to control for sources of variation in data in search of parsimony. The degree of control that can be applied in any analysis is dependent on the study design, nature of the data and familiarity with the issues of dynamics of human behaviour. The purpose of this chapter is to re-introduce the issue of control in a practical setting and to illustrate the benefits gained as a result of incorporating control within the analytical framework. To demonstrate this, we begin with the simplest analysis commonly known as bivariate analysis where the relationship between an explanatory variable and an outcome is explored. The main issue with such exploratory data analyses is that we would ignore the influence of other variables on the outcome that may be operating through the selected explanatory variable (e.g. see Figure 1.3). In other words, we will need to formally allow for control in the analysis. In this chapter, we illustrate the process of building in control in the analysis. The example used in this chapter is survival in old age. Death is an inevitable outcome of old age given natural processes, yet some people die soon after retirement while others may survive to ripe old age. An obvious question would be what factors may explain the variation in death (or survival) post-retirement. On the other hand, due to a heterogeneous survivor population, defining the outcome as surviving or dying may not be sensitive enough to distinguish random effects from systematic effects of some quality of life variables. Therefore we may increase complexity in the analyses by modelling a multinomial categorical response variable (survivor and in community, survivor and in care, died) and by modeling duration survived. Therefore, in this chapter we work through the steps of applying progressively more complex methodologies for the analysis of survival in old age, highlighting issues of control, and interpreting and discussing the results. In the final sections (2.7 and 2.8) we compare and contrast the benefits and drawbacks of the different methodologies.

2.2. BACKGROUND

Shahtahmasebi and Wenger ([32], also see [2, 33]) argue that the types of factors found to be associated with survival in old age have reflected, in large part, the particular research disciplines informing the various studies. For example, one US researcher has concluded that 'there is no single factor which determines longevity but rather a constellation of biological, psychological and social factors amounting to an elite status' [34]. He found that people with high intelligence, sound financial status, good health and intact marriages may expect to live longer. A study of US working class elderly similarly found that being female, coupled with the competent performance of daily routines, was the best discriminator for short-term survival [35].

In a UK study, Abrams [36] looked at cross-tabulations of potential explanatory variables by survival/non-survival and found that survival in the 65-69 age group was related to being female, being in good health and having low levels of loneliness, depression, sensory impairment and anxiety and having high levels of social interaction, life satisfaction, morale, activity and integration. However, the interactions between these variables were not explored.

Work by Wenger [2] on the basis of 1979-1983 data suggested that there may be a degree of association between the variables shown in Table 2.1 and the outcome variable 'deceased/alive'. Death was found to be more common amongst those who were older, male (in all age groups), widowed, in poor health (as perceived by the respondents), restricted in mobility, working class, on lower incomes, tenants, living alone or with younger relatives, frequently in contact with relatives and/or isolated. The last two items represent both ends of a spectrum and many old people had levels of contact between these extremes. For women, death was more common amongst those with many children and the lonely; for men, death was more common amongst those with low morale. It can be seen that these variables are inter-related. For instance, with death rates higher for men in all age groups, more women are widowed and living alone. Marital status and household composition, therefore, are not independent of gender. By the same token, health and restricted mobility are inter-related, as are social class, income and home tenure [35, 37].

The above findings, in general, are in agreement with other studies [38-48]. Higher levels of occupation, class, income and/or education are indicators of socio-economic status and appear to be associated with lower morbidity and mortality. Conversely, bereavement (usually, widowhood) [43, 49, 50], no supportive network and social isolation [41, 51] are reported to be associated with higher morbidity and mortality rates. Clearly a large number of factors have been suggested as being associated with survival.

2.3. DATA DESCRIPTION AND EXPLORATORY ANALYSES

The data for this chapter came from the NWEP (Section 1.5), a large social survey questionnaire which was designed to explore the lives of elderly people living in rural areas. The questionnaire covered topics such as personal details, housing, health, dependency and mobility, domiciliary and social services, informal support and contact with relatives/neighbours/friends. Survey questionnaires and observational studies frequently use different types of measurement within the same study structure e.g. scales or scoring systems to measure loneliness or morale, subjective measures such as self-reported health and perception of neighbourhood. There are consequences and implications for the analysis which will be discussed in this chapter and throughout this book.

As shown in Figure 1.6, in 1983 and 1987 the survey traced all respondents who were alive and took part in the survey in 1979. Initially our interest was in the rate of survival therefore all those who were still alive in 1987 were coded as survivors and the remainder were coded as deceased thus creating a binary outcome variable with two categories (survivor/deceased or 1/0). This variable is the **outcome variable** 'survival'. A number of explanatory variables was extracted from the database (see Appendix I). For a meaningful cross-classification with **the outcome variable** 'survival', explanatory variables must also be categorical. However, care must be taken when categorising variables. Data collected in a survey questionnaire may include variables such as 'household composition', 'home tenure' or 'marital status' which may not have sufficient numbers in some of the categories due to the small sample size thus requiring re-categorisation. In practice, categorisation depends on the nature of the variable being analysed and a degree of common sense. For example, for ordinal variables such as age and income the categorisation would be based on a priori, or, to re-categorise an ordinal variable then the category with the smallest cell frequency should be combined with its adjacent category. In the current analysis, for variables with a large number of categories, adjacent categories were cobined in order to reduce the number of categories. The merging of categories helped to reduce the problem of small cell frequencies in the cross-tabulations.

Less than one percent of the cases had missing values for most variables and we adopted the simple 'imputation' strategy of allocating such cases to the variable categories with the highest frequency. However, there were rather more missing observations for variables such as income, number in network, morale, isolation measure, and loneliness measure. For income, fieldwork experience indicated that the majority of refusals were from higher income respondents and all were therefore allocated to the upper income category. A separate non-response category was retained for the remaining variables.

After data preparation, we cross-tabulated the explanatory variables with the survival variable in two-way contingency tables. To explore the relationship between the explanatory variables and survival in old age, we used the Pearson chi-squared test statistic (χ^2) and its associated p-value from the contingency tables. The results are shown in Table 2.1. Most of the variables examined were significantly related to survival in old age. Over 60% of the variables were significant at the 5% level and a further three variables at the 10% level: these were social class, morale and loneliness measure. From the percentages in each category we could explore the nature of the relationship with survival. For example, survival decreased with age and females were expected to live longer than males; those who classified themselves as British had a higher survival rate along with owner occupiers, those in higher income brackets and those in good health.

It is possible that some of these variables owe their significance to their association with age. To explore how strongly the explanatory variables may be interrelated, we calculated the Cramer's υ measure of association for all the variables in the analysis. These results are shown in Table 2.2 which confirms that there are complex patterns of inter-relationships between the explanatory variables. Due to the small sample size, **a Cramer's υ of over 0.2 was** considered to indicate a strong association. For example, household composition was associated with marital status, number of children, income, relative seen most often, frequency of contact with family, network type, hours spent alone, isolation and loneliness. However, these variables themselves are interrelated with each other, as well as with other variables in the table. For example, network type is correlated with hours spent alone, isolation, loneliness, morale, health and visits from the doctor. Therefore, it would be unwise to infer causal effects from Table 2.1. In other words, given the results in Table 2.2, we cannot conclude a direct and independent relationship between each explanatory variable in Table 2.1 and survival. Thus, the question to be asked is whether household composition and network type, which are significant in Table 2.1, reflect social determinants of survival in old age, or whether network type is merely acting as a proxy for age, dependency or health effects. A multivariate analysis is therefore required to allow us to make conclusions about the effect of each explanatory variable on survival, having controlled for other explanatory variables.

Table 2.1. Cross-classification of 'survival' variable with some explanatory variables (% survived in each category)(goodness of fit is based on the Pearson χ^2, *p≤0.05, **p≤0.01, ***p≤0.001), N=524

Demographic variables	% survived		% survived		% survived
Age***		Gender*		Household composition*	
65-74	70	male	51	lives alone	55
75-79	49	female	61	with spouse	66
80+	33			with other	51
Marital status*		Number of children		Arrival age in community*	
single	57	no children	59	long-term	52
married	64	1	62	middle-age mover	69
widowed	52	2	49	retirement mover	50
		3	61	retirement migrant	62
		4+	56		
Ethnicity*					
English	53				
Welsh	56				
½ Welsh	50				
British	87				
Other	67				
Social variables					
No. in network		Relative seen most often		Frequency of contact with family	
small	56	children	53	daily	55
medium	56	sibling	60	weekly	63
large	63		57	monthly	60
		nephew/niece/cousin			
missing	43	other	60	less often	50
Network type**		Hours spent alone			
family dependent	44	up to 6 hours	59		

locally integrated	59	more than 6 hours	55		
local self-contained	59				
wider community focused	71				
private restricted	58				
Socio-economic variables					
Income*		Social class+		Home tenure**	
up to £59	52	middle	62	owner	64
£60-99	64	skilled	55	rent	52
£100+ per week	65	semi-/unskilled	50	other	45
Health and dependency variables					
Visit from doctor*		Health ltd. activities***		Visit from dist. nurse***	
yes	46	yes, limited activities	66	yes	38
no	61	no, not limited	49	no	61
Self-assessed health***		Have home help**		Have private home help*	
excellent/good	71	yes	32	yes	41
alright for age	50	no	59	no	59
fair	46				
poor	14				
Quality of life variables					
Isolation measure		Loneliness measure		Morale	
not isolated	62	not lonely	62	low	46
moderately isolated	55	moderately lonely	55	medium	57
very isolated	48	very lonely	42	high morale	61
missing	41	missing	43	missing	44
Self-assessed loneliness*		Worry over bills			
feels lonely	51	worry	58		
does not feel lonely	60	do not worry	56		

Table 2.1 informs us that there are significant relationships between the outcome and the explanatory variables. Furthermore, the values highlighted in bold in Table 2.2 suggest a degree of multicollinearity. As explained in the introduction, this means that the relationship between survival and an explanatory variable (e.g. network type) may be influenced by the relationship between that factor (network type) and other explanatory variables e.g. the dependency variables. As was shown in Figure 1.3, we are interested in the net effect of explanatory variables on survival in old age. In examining the net effect of an explanatory variable on the response, we must 'control' for the effect of other explanatory variables.

One way of imposing 'control' is through the method of disaggregation i.e. multi-way cross-tabulations of the outcome, survival in this case, with two or more explanatory variables. There are several problems with such an approach. First, it is an extension of the two-way cross-classification process and will produce numerous tables to examine and interpret. In studies of this type, where a large number of variables is involved, the examination and interpretation of a large number of tables will be cumbersome, painstaking and speculative, and the interpretation of such tables may lead to unsatisfactory conclusions. Second, multi-way cross-tabulation may lead to (very) small cell frequencies which can not be interpreted in a meaningful way. Third, this method gives a jagged picture of the data because it will not allow the smoothing out of continuous variables e.g. age will have to be categorised. Furthermore, this method provides no way of quantifying and of testing for the statistical significance of the effects of each explanatory variable.

2.4. STATISTICAL MODELLING OF BINARY SURVIVAL IN OLD AGE

The analysis seeks to explore the pattern of association between explanatory variables and survival to the end of the project 'window'. The nature of the data set and the availability of the outcome variables at the two time points (1983 and 1987) means that other analyses are also possible. For example, the 1983 outcome may be modelled with the explanatory variables from the 1979 survey questionnaire. Similarly, survival of those aged over 75 after 4 and 8 years can be modelled (see [32]). However, for the sake of illustration, we only present the results from the analysis of the 1987 outcome with 1979 explanatory variables. For the full analysis see [28, 33].

Cases with missing values for the response variables (around 2%) were dropped from the analyses. Explanatory variables with missing values were treated as described in Section 2.3. In other words, those explanatory variables with the proportion of missing values of up to 1% were re-categorised. A separate 'missing' category was created for explanatory variables with more than 1% of values missing.

Assume that y, the response variable 'survivor (1)/non-survivor (0)' can be expressed as a function of a set of explanatory variables. For the ith individual, we have

$$y_i = \beta x_i + \varepsilon_i$$

In operationalizing this model with a binary response, the probability of survival is assumed to be a logistic function of explanatory variables i.e. the standard logistic transformation is used (see Appendix II.I):

$$p(y=1, \text{survival}|x) = \frac{\exp\beta xp}{1+\exp\beta xp}$$

Table 2.2. Measures of association (Cramer's v) between the 1979 explanatory variables as listed in Table 2.1 (N=524). Values greater than 0.2 indicate association

Variables	1	2	3	4	5	6	7	8	9	10	11	12	13	14	15	16	17	18	19	20	21	22	23	24	25	26
Demographic Variables																										
1. Age		0.15	0.22	0.23	0.09	0.13	0.13	0.18	0.11	0.11	0.11	0.13	0.12	0.18	0.13	0.15	0.12	0.12	0.11	0.07	0.14	0.20	0.27	0.20	0.20	0.18
2. Gender		-	0.31	0.36	0.10	0.03	0.02	0.23	0.05	0.05	0.07	0.09	0.12	0.08	0.24	0.26	0.10	0.08	0.14	0.08	0.12	0.14	0.00	0.07	0.01	0.02
3. Household composition			-	0.60	0.23	0.14	0.12	0.27	0.08	0.14	0.20	0.60	0.12	0.30	0.75	0.52	0.16	0.11	0.30	0.04	0.07	0.01	0.04	0.10	0.13	0.12
4. Marital status				-	0.45	0.11	0.08	0.29	0.04	0.09	0.35	0.10	0.11	0.19	0.56	0.42	0.12	0.08	0.33	0.06	0.10	0.07	0.11	0.13	0.04	0.05
5. No. children					-	0.12	0.08	0.13	0.13	0.17	0.44	0.17	0.10	0.16	0.19	0.18	0.11	0.07	0.42	0.15	0.09	0.09	0.08	0.06	0.13	0.07
6. Arrival age						-	0.32	0.14	0.16	0.12	0.11	0.14	0.09	0.26	0.14	0.14	0.15	0.09	0.12	0.04	0.05	0.09	0.08	0.07	0.06	0.07
7. Ethnicity							-	0.16	0.16	0.15	0.11	0.18	0.12	0.26	0.13	0.09	0.14	0.12	0.11	0.03	0.15	0.07	0.03	0.11	0.10	0.13
Socio-economic Variables																										
8. Income								-	0.22	0.21	0.12	0.11	0.15	0.15	0.28	0.24	0.30	0.13	0.11	0.14	0.11	0.09	0.07	0.07	0.05	0.07
9. Social class									-	0.27	0.11	0.11	0.10	0.16	0.09	0.16	0.10	0.10	0.07	0.19	0.10	0.03	0.03	0.07	0.13	0.16
10. Home tenure										-	0.10	0.17	0.11	0.19	0.12	0.19	0.16	0.16	0.11	0.11	0.12	0.12	0.19	0.04	0.08	0.05
Social Variables																										
11. Relative seen											-	0.23	0.15	0.21	0.22	0.24	0.18	0.12	0.10	0.14	0.11	0.08	0.06	0.11	0.09	0.03
12. Frequency of contact												-	0.14	0.35	0.35	0.23	0.15	0.08	0.15	0.03	0.07	0.04	0.71	0.03	0.14	0.16
13. Network size													-	0.29	0.20	0.49	0.48	0.36	0.18	0.23	0.11	0.06	0.04	0.05	0.17	0.10
14. Network type														-	0.25	0.23	0.24	0.24	0.23	0.16	0.18	0.24	0.20	0.19	0.16	0.05
15.															-	0.67	0.36	0.20	0.36	0.05	0.10	0.03	0.03	0.08	0.08	0.12

Variables	1	2	3	4	5	6	7	8	9	10	11	12	13	14	15	16	17	18	19	20	21	22	23	24	25	26
Hours alone																										
Quality-of-life Variables																										
16. Isolation measure																-	0.41	0.38	0.38	0.33	0.15	0.13	0.12	0.18	0.23	0.18
17. Loneliness measure																	-	0.48	0.46	0.20	0.33	0.20	0.09	0.21	0.15	0.12
18. Morale																		-	0.48	0.30	0.30	0.35	0.16	0.17	0.19	0.13
19. Loneliness																			-	0.20	0.33	0.20	0.09	0.21	0.15	0.12
20. Worry bills																				-	0.19	0.10	0.08	0.11	0.08	0.00
Health and Dependency Variables																										
21. Health status																					-	0.56	0.20	0.20	0.23	0.09
22. Health limit																						-	0.19	0.17	0.13	0.07
23. Doctor																							-	0.34	0.18	0.12
24. District nurse																								-	0.24	0.14
25. Home help																									-	0.08
26. Private help																										-

variable selection and model criticism is based on likelihood ratio test statistic (χ^2). Although we used the statistical software package GLIM [52] for model fitting, any standard statistical package such as Minitab, Genstat, SAS, SABRE, LIMDEP, NLOGIT and STATA may be used to fit a logistic model. Other transformations e.g. the probit and the complementary log-log are also possible and applicable, and can easily be carried out in GLIM.

2.4.1. Variable Selection

When dealing with a large number of variables, it is more convenient to automate the variable selection process by writing a macro or procedure to carry out the steps involved in the selection process, be it forward or backward selection. However, there are advantages in performing the selection process manually, as we have done. Because of the large number of variables, a 'forward' iterative method of variable selection was adopted. First, we construct as many models as the number of explanatory variables and compare these models using the likelihood ratio test statistic (χ^2), see Table 2.3. The best fitting model is selected, and the explanatory variable which is most significant at the 5% level is included in the model. Variable selection proceeds with the remaining variables being considered for inclusion in the model. For example, from Table 2.3, 'age' is the most significant variable, so this is included in the best fitting model. Variable selection continues with 'constant + age' as Model 1, and variables with a significance level higher than 5% such as 'household composition', 'marital status', 'income' are dropped from the analysis. The process continues until all significant variables are included in the final model and there are no variables remaining significant at the 5% level. This approach can be very instructive in an exploratory study. In particular, a marked change in the significance of a remaining variable when a new variable is added to the model is indicative of a spurious relationship arising from statistical association with the added variable. On the other hand, with high multicollinearity in the data, the final model may be heavily dependent upon a marginal choice between two variables at some stage in the model-building process. It is important to detect when this is occurring in order to prevent undue emphasis being placed on one variable when others are practically indistinguishable in their explanatory power. Moreover, identification of nearly interchangeable variables may guide further research in reducing multicollinearity problems by combining variables to form composite indices.

Here we are concerned with assessing the *prima facie* evidence of the relationship between social characteristics and longevity in old age. The statistical modelling approach we have adopted seeks to achieve this objective by identifying *ceteris paribus* the systematic relationships between the explanatory variables and survival, distinguishing these relationships from the irregular, random variations in the data on the one hand, and the misleading effects of multicollinearity on the other.

As shown in Table 2.3, there are 18 variables which appear to be significantly related to survival on their own. Once age, sex and self-assessed health are entered in the model, there are only six variables which remain statistically significant at the 5% level. Out of these, only the variables 'arrival age', 'visits from district nurse' and 'ethnicity' are accepted in the final model. The model fitting results for this analysis are shown in Table 2.4.

A specific example of multicollinearity is provided by the variables 'self-assessed health' and 'health limited activities'. These two variables appear to be significantly related to survival on their own ($\chi^2=33.0$ and $\chi^2=15.9$ respectively). However, when controlling for 'age' and 'self-assessed health', 'health limited activities' ceases to be significant ($\chi^2=0.1$). In this instance, the inclusion of 'health limited activities' does not make a significant contribution towards explaining the variation in survival once age and state of health have been controlled for. This becomes clearer when testing for the effect of 'state of health' while controlling for 'health limited activities'. The inclusion of 'health' in the model leads to 'health limited activities' becoming non-significant ($\chi^2=0.2$). So there is no need to proceed with an alternative model which includes 'health limited activities' in parallel with the model which includes 'state of health'. Both variables measure the same effect (dependency due to ill health) and, in this case, 'state of health' appears to be a better predictor and fully controls for the effects of 'health limited activities'. This initial result suggests a correlation between 'age', 'self-assessed health', and 'health limited activities'.

In practice, when selecting a model, it is not uncommon to encounter an ambiguity problem. This means situations in which, after fitting models, the resulting p-values for the effects of two explanatory variables are very small or sufficiently close that we are unable to distinguish a dominant effect. Under such circumstances, alternative models should be constructed which may lead to the examination and interpretation of more than one parsimonious model.

2.4.2. Interpretation

To explore fully the effect of each explanatory variable on the model of survival, alternative restricted models are compared with the full model. This is done by dropping an explanatory variable from the full model, observing the change in the model deviance and then putting it back in the model. This process is repeated for all the variables which are in the full model. The full model fitting results are shown in Table 2.4, which also shows the likelihood ratio test statistic (χ^2) for each restricted model and its respective associated p-value. A further feature of this method is the facility to calculate the survival probabilities (or alternatively odds ratios) for each explanatory variable *ceteris paribus*. For example, we can estimate the death (failure) rate from the sample as shown in Appendix II.II. For example, those who claimed to be in a fair or poor state of health are 0.75 times as likely to survive than those who claimed to be in a good state of health (Appendix II.II).

For this first round of analysis of survival in old age, we have presented the results in Table 2.4 in order to provide an understanding of the effect of each explanatory variable included in the model. When the analysis is more exploratory in nature, it is desirable to examine the effect that each explanatory variable may have on the final model. For example, as shown in Table 2.4, parameter estimates and test statistics for the full model can be compared with those from a series of restricted models excluding a single variable from the model. Table 2.4 displays the change in likelihood ratio from the full model to a restricted model which has a chi-squared distribution and its associated p-value. However, it is interesting to note what happens to the parameter estimates as each variable is dropped from the model. The age effect is clear: probability of survival decreases with increasing age. This effect does not appear to interact with or be influenced by other variables; its parameter estimate hardly changes over the restricted models. Similarly, females appear to live longer. Although it can be noticed that the sex effect is reduced when health status and age are dropped from the model, there is a drop in its parameter estimate when health status is dropped from the model. The largest reduction in the sex effect occurs when age is dropped from the model (0.24). This indicates that the survival rate of females is clearly dependent on their age and state of health. We can see that age also has an impact on state of health for those who claimed to be 'alright for age'. Those who claimed to be in receipt of district nurse services have a lower likelihood of survival. This result does not imply that district nurse services reduce the survival rate of the elderly! It can be seen from the restricted models that both 'age' and 'state of health' have an influence on this variable. Our data and experience suggest that those elderly who are more dependent and in poor health are more likely to receive visits from the district nurse. This is a causality problem where an impending event causes a reaction, i.e. impending death causes visits from the district nurse. Indeed, visits from the district nurse become more likely and frequent in the weeks and months preceding death. Finally, the 'arrival age in community' effect does not appear to be affected by 'ethnicity', but ethnicity appears to be affected by 'arrival age in community' and possibly age. The 'arrival age in community' may be affected by age. The parameter estimates of both retired movers and retired migrants have decreased by 0.2 and 0.37 respectively when age is excluded from the model. Although 'arrival age in community' may be acting as a proxy for the age effect, when age is excluded from the model, in the final model both 'arrival age in community' and 'ethnicity' are statistically significant. However, when 'arrival age in community' is excluded from the model, the most noticeable effects are on the parameter estimates of those who claimed to be Welsh and half-Welsh. These two groups may be long term residents or those who move after retirement to be close to their children. On the other hand, those who claimed to be British appear mostly to be of middle class background. On the whole, the changes in the parameter estimates are relatively small, indicating that the variables may be direct and independent effects on survival. It is straightforward to test for interaction effects such as the 'arrival age in community' by 'ethnicity' effect. In a larger data set, this would be as simple as creating a dummy variable for the interaction term e.g. middle aged movers who are British or retired movers who are Welsh, and including it in the full model. It must be noted that the interaction terms must be related to the main effects already present in the full model [53]. In this case, both variables 'arrival age in community' and 'ethnicity' are statistically significant and are present in the full model.

2.4.3. Summary

It was illustrated that cross-tabulations are simple and easy to carry out. When such an exploratory analysis is combined with hypothesis testing using the chi-squared test statistic, cross-tabulations would serve as a useful initial step in getting an idea about the data. However, the results from a cross-tabulation are of meagre value if taken as independent inferential statements. This is due to lack of any control; when investigating the relationship between the response and each explanatory variable, the effects of other variables must be controlled for. In this first round of analysis, we demonstrated the application of statistical modelling to disentangle the complex relationships among the variables. Specifically, with statistical modelling we were able to address the following:-

i. exploration of the relationship between survival and each explanatory variable in the presence of other factors i.e. control for other effects, thus identifying the systematic effects;
ii. exploration of the relationships between explanatory variables (multicollinearity) e.g. the relationships between 'age', 'sex', 'self-assessed health' and 'health limited activities';
iii. estimation and quantification of the effect of explanatory variables on survival in terms of probabilities, thereby enabling *ceteris paribus* conclusions about the effect of each explanatory variable on survival;
iv. the large number of explanatory variables thought to be related to survival is reduced to a few factors which are easy to manage and interpret.

Table 2.3. List of Explanatory Variables from 1979 and initial model fitting results for the logistic regression of survival/non-survival, response variable = outcome 1987, N= 524

Explanatory variables	Chi-sq+	d.f
Age	60.1*	1
Sex	4.6*	1
Household composition	9.1	4
Marital status	7.7	3
Morale	7.1	3
Income	10.6*	3
Housing tenure	15.3*	2
Number of children	0.6	1
Relative seen most	6.0	4
Frequency see family	5.3	3
Arrival age in community†	9.9*	3
Number in support network†	4.7	3
Ever feel lonely	9.4	5
Network type†	15.4*	4
State of health	33.0*	2
Health limited activities	15.9*	1
Do you get angry any more	12.7*	2
Visit from doctor in last 6 months‡	8.7*	1
Visit from health visitor in the last 6 months‡	3.6	1
Visit from district nurse in the last 6 months ‡	16.7*	1
Hours alone in the house	4.8	3
Alone in the house (nights)	5.7*	1
Worry over bills	7.9*	3
Isolation measure†	3.4	1
Loneliness measure†	6.4*	1
Number of elderly in the house	0.8	1
Social class	10.7*	2
Home help	11.0*	1
Private home help	5.2*	1
Ethnicity	15.9*	4

+ Likelihood ratio test showing the effect of each variable on its own in the logistic model.
* Variables significant at the 5% level.
† See Appendix I.
‡ Binary dummy variables, see Appendix I (also see Table 2.1).

Table 2.4. Model fitting results for logistic regression of survival/non-survival: comparison of the parameter estimates of the selected model, response variable= outcome 1987, N=524

Effect	Full Model	No Nurse Effect	No Arrival Effect	No Sex Effect	No Health Effect	No Age Effect	No Ethnicity Effect
Age	-0.11	-0.12	-0.11	-0.10	-0.12		-0.11
Sex							
Male	0.00	0.00	0.00		0.00	0.00	0.00
Female	0.85 (0.23)	0.82	0.82		0.74	0.61	0.85
State of health							
Excellent/good	0.00	0.00	0.00	0.00		0.00	0.00
Alright	-0.72 (0.60)	-0.76	-0.71	-0.63		-0.90	-0.74
Fair/poor	-1.24 (0.75)	-1.32	-1.10	-1.13		-1.25	-1.24
District nurse							
No	0.00		0.00	0.00	0.00	0.00	0.00
Yes	-0.62 (0.57)		-0.60	-0.54	-0.78	-0.89	-0.62
Arrival age in community							
Long-term resident	0.00	0.00		0.00	0.00	0.00	0.00
Middle aged mover	0.86 (0.23)	0.86		0.85	0.77	0.77	0.83
Retired mover	0.16 (0.38)	0.22		0.17	0.10	-0.04	0.17
Retired migrant	0.89 (0.23)	0.90		0.74	0.80	0.52	0.80
Ethnicity							
English	0.00	0.00	0.00	0.00	0.00	0.00	
Welsh	0.35 (0.33)	0.39	-0.11	0.35	0.33	0.37	
Half Welsh	0.02 (0.41)	0.12	-0.42	-0.03	-0.08	0.05	
British	1.65 (0.12)	1.69	1.53	1.65	1.60	1.82	
Other	0.54 (0.29)	0.48	0.32	0.49	0.61	0.78	
Log-likelihood	-293.8	-296.36	-300.5	-302.08	-305.3	-318.5	-298.6
Likelihood ratio χ^2		5.1	13.3	16.6	23	49.4	9.5
D.F.		1	3	1	2	1	4
P		0.025	0.004	0.00005	0.00001	0.00001	0.05

Note: Values in brackets show probability of death over eight years assuming a sample death rate of 40% over the project window, see Appendix I.

2.5. STATISTICAL MODELLING OF MULTINOMIAL SURVIVAL IN OLD AGE

So far we have investigated the probability of being a survivor (or deceased) after eight years for an elderly individual in the sample. We did this in the previous section by combining together all survivors, regardless of their degree of frailty, as one category and all deceased, regardless of when they died during the project window, as another category. However, in old age, the 'path' to death could be viewed as a sequential process as shown in Figure 2.1. All individuals were alive and in the community at the start of the project. Over the subsequent years, some became dependent before death and some were still in the community. One outcome that could be used to measure dependency prior to death is entry into residential care. Therefore it is reasonable to distinguish between two types of survivor: survivors in the community and survivors in residential care. Such a distinction provides a more detailed, and potentially more insightful, response variable of survival in old age and makes more use of the data available. The outcome now has three possible events: survivor in the community, survivor in residential care and deceased. Clearly, the logistic regression applied in the previous section is no longer appropriate. This section concentrates on the application of a more complex family of multinomial response models for ordered outcome processes.

Figure 2.1 Possible outcomes over the project window

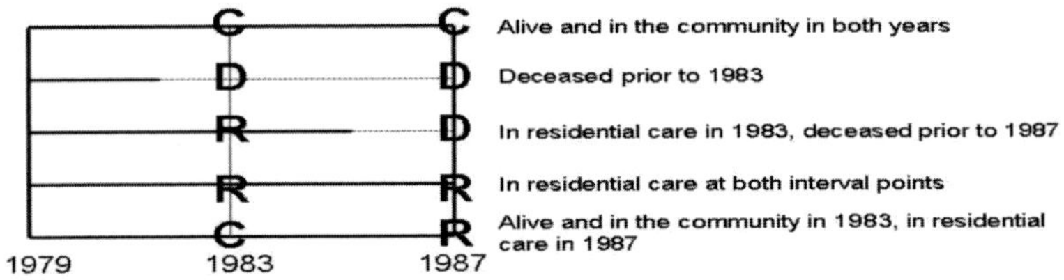

```
           C        C     Alive and in the community in both years
           D        D     Deceased prior to 1983
           R        D     In residential care in 1983, deceased prior to 1987
           R        R     In residential care at both interval points
           C        R     Alive and in the community in 1983, in residential
                          care in 1987
   1979   1983     1987
```

2.5.1. Statistical Approach and Assumptions

Here we observe three possible outcomes in the process of survival in old age. Such multinomial response data can be modelled in several ways, two of which are:

- To construct a set of binary dummy variable(s) which will include one category (1) against other categories (0) for each of the outcomes. Analysis could then be performed using binary logistic regression as demonstrated, in the previous section (also see [23, 24]).
- To specify and fit a general multinomial model to the data. This means that the response has three or more possible outcomes each of which has a non-zero probability of occurring (see Appendix III).

2.5.2. Model Specification

All the elderly respondents in the project were alive and in the community at the start of the project. Some elderly respondents entered residential care, and some died. As illustrated in Figure 2.1 we can assume sequential ordinality in the three response categories ('in the community', 'in care' and 'deceased') leading to a special case of the multinomial response model. This is equivalent to assuming some latent variable which measures the degree of dependence or frailty (see Figure 2.2); at high levels of this latent variable, individuals are expected to be in the community but when they cross over some threshold of dependence they would enter residential care. Lower levels of this variable are associated with death. In other words, we could regard the latent variable in two ways: first, as a dependency measure; second, as an indicator of the strength of independence of an individual. The lower the independence, the greater are the levels of dependency and the higher is the chance of death.

Individuals with identical observed characteristics may have different outcomes (e.g one may be in the community, another in residential care) because of the unobserved variables and elements of chance in the factors involved. The model is operationalized in terms of the probabilities of outcomes to allow for these uncertainties (see Appendix III). However, the formal latent variable formulation permits us to quantify the effect of specific factors on the probability of different outcomes.

We proceed by assuming the probability of an individual falling in any of the response categories to be a logit function of the explanatory variables, see Appendix III.

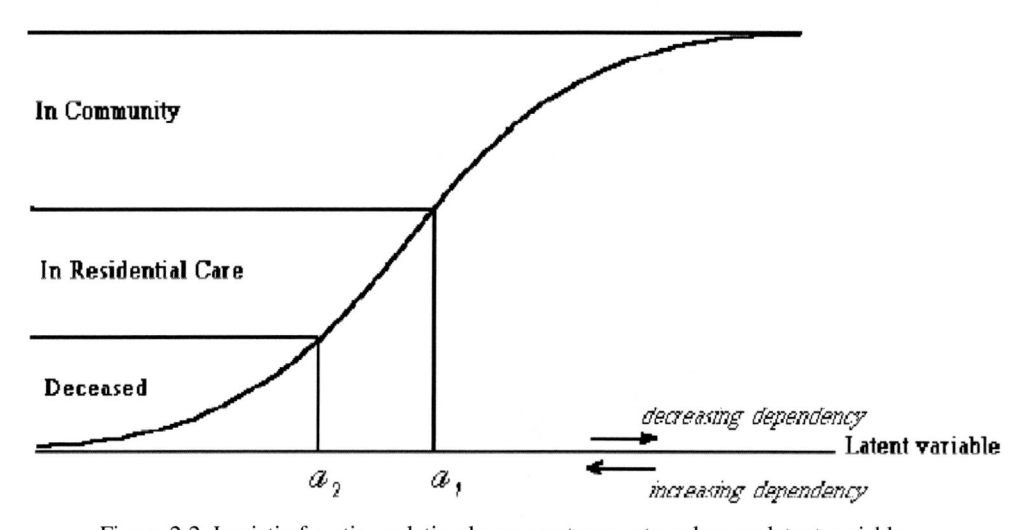

Figure 2.2. Logistic function relating known outcomes to unknown latent variable.

The formulation for the ordered multinomial model (see Appendix III) is demonstrated in Figure 2.2. The 'latent' variable in this formulation is given by the response y: if $y_i > \alpha_1$ there is survival in the community, if $\alpha_2 < y_i \leq \alpha_1$ there is entry into residential care, and if $y_i \leq \alpha_2$ then death. Other ordinal specifications are possible [54], but the approach adopted here has the advantage of needing only a single linear predictor (see also [55]).

To operationalize this model, the likelihood method of inference was used for parameter estimation. FORTRAN programs were developed to cope with routine algebra/matrix calculations involved with the likelihood estimation, likelihood ratio statistic (χ^2) and associated p-values. However, nowadays such a model may be fitted to data routinely within major statistical software packages. As will be seen in Chapter 5, SABRE can easily be used.

2.5.3. Variable Selection

Variable selection proceeds exactly as before. We used a forward iterative variable selection method in which variables were entered in the model one at a time and their effects, based on the χ^2 test statistic, were noted. The variable with the largest χ^2 and smallest p-value was selected for inclusion in the model first and the model-building process then continued until no further variables left out of the model were significant at the 5% level. The results were then checked for the possibility of alternative models e.g. where the difference between two effects may be too small to be distinguishable or where practical significance took priority over statistical significance. There were no causes for concern. The list of variables and model fitting results are shown in tables 2.5 and 2.6 respectively.

Table 2.5. List of Explanatory Variables from 1979 and initial model fitting results, response variable = outcome 1987, N=524

Explanatory variables	Chi-sq+	d.f
Age	74.7*	1
Sex	3.3*	1
Household composition††	9.4*	2
Marital status††	10.9*	2
Morale	9.0*	3
Income††	10.8*	2
House tenure	12.7*	2
Number of children	0.1	1
Relative seen most††	3.3	3
Frequency see family	1.4	3
Arrival age in community†	9.9*	3
Number in support network†	3.7	2
Ever feel lonely††	5.3*	1
Network type†	14.5*	4
State of health	34.5*	2
Health limited activities	15.5*	1
Do you get angry any more	6.0*	2
Visit from doctor in last 6 months‡	11.5*	1
Visit health visitor in last 6 months	5.9*	1
Visit district nurse in last 6 months ‡	18.3*	1
Hours alone in the house††	1.4	1
Alone in the house (nights)	1.1	1
Worry over bills††	0.7	1
Isolation measure†	8.4*	1
Loneliness measure†	7.9*	1
Number of elderly in the house	0.9	1
Social class	6.9*	2
Home help	14.7*	1
Private home help	5.9*	1
Ethnicity	16.0*	4

+ Likelihood ratio test statistic showing the effect of each variable on its own in the logit model.
* Variables significant at 5% level when on their own.
† See Appendix I for variable definition.
‡ Binary dummy variables
†† some categories in these variables were collapsed in order to maintain reasonable cell frequencies.

Table 2.6. Results for three-category (in the community, in residential care, deceased) response model, response variable = outcome 1987, N = 524

Explanatory variables	Full Model parameter estimates	L.R χ2	d.f	p
Age	-0.13	76.1	1	«0.00001
Sex		14.7	1	0.0001
Male	0.00			
Female	0.76			
State of health		29.8	2	<0.0001
Excellent/good	0.00			
All right for age	-0.76			
Fair/poor	-1.31			
Arrival age in community		15.7	3	0.0013
Long-term resident	0.00			
Middle aged mover	0.80			
Retirement mover	0.19			
Retirement migrant	0.80			
α1	-9.4			
α2	-9.7			
Log-likelihood	-388.1			

2.5.4. Interpretation

The interpretation can be assisted by the probability curve in Figure 2.2. The probability of a latent variable value between α_1 and α_2 specifies the probability of an individual being in residential care, below α_2 indicates the probability of death for an individual with the same age; and above α_2 indicates the probability of remaining in the community. Table 2.6 only provides an indication of the direction of the effect, e.g. a negative effect implies a lower probability of survival and a positive effect implies a higher probability of survival. The rationale behind Figure 2.2 was used to construct Figures 2.3-2.5. These figures show plots of cumulative probabilities for different effects against age with other variables set to their reference category values as appropriate. The probability of going into care is represented by the area (R) between the areas representing probability of survival in the community (C) and probability of death (D). The results from Table 2.6 were substituted into equations (1)-(3) (see Appendix III) to estimate these probabilities. Including interactions in the model would have provided a more flexible specification but this was not possible due to the limited size of these data.

As would be expected, Table 2.6 indicates that the older the respondents, the less likelihood of survival in the community and that female respondents are more likely to survive in the community. It can be seen from Figure 2.3 that the probability of survival in the community after eight years (1979-87, from Table 2.6) for those who are a male, in good/excellent health, and a long-term resident decreases from 0.48 at age 73, to 0.35 at 77, and to 0.24 at age 81 (remember that the youngest member of the sample was 65 in 1979).

However, while the probability of death is monotone increasing (i.e. from 1.0- 0.55=0.45 at age 73, to 1.0-0.42=0.58 at 77, and to 1.0-0.30=0.70 at 81), the probability of being in care appears to be fairly constant (i.e. from 0.55-0.48=0.07 at age 73, to 0.42-0.35=0.07 at age 77, and to 0.30- 0.24=0.06 at 81).

Because of the importance of age, it was used as a 'base' when considering other effects. The variable sex is significant. To see how elderly males compare with elderly females, the results from Table 2.6 were substituted into formulae (1) and (2) in Appendix III controlling for age. The resulting probabilities were used to construct the probability diagrams shown in Figures 2.4 (a) and (b). By comparing Figure 2.4(a) with Figure 2.4(b), the differences between men and women can be explored. For instance, at the age of 73, women are about 38% (0.66/0.48=1.38) more likely to remain in the community than men. Women appear to be more likely to survive longer in the community and hence may enter into care at an older age. Using such a decomposition we proceed with the interpretation of the remaining effects.

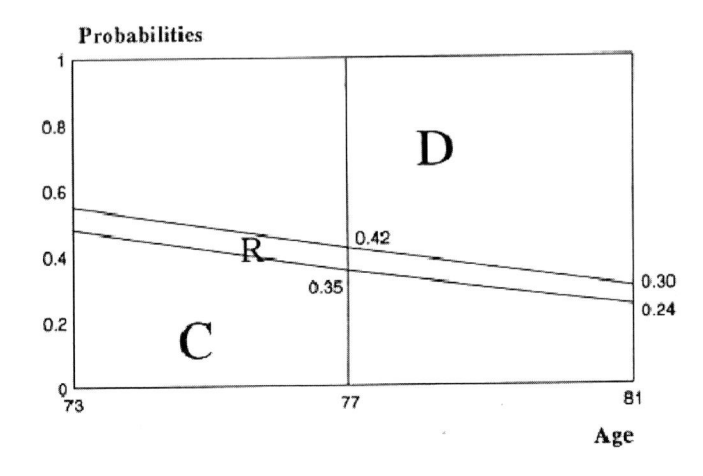

Figure 2.3. Diagrammatical representation of the multinomial response probability distribution given observed age.

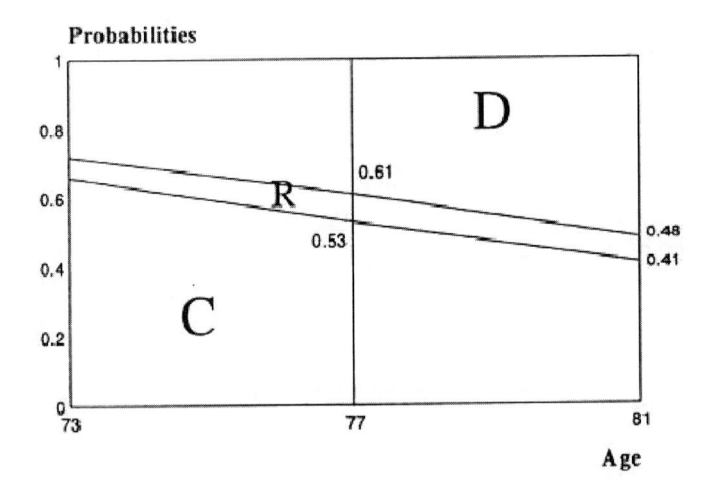

2.4(a) multinomial probability of survival of a female for observed age, from Table 2.6.

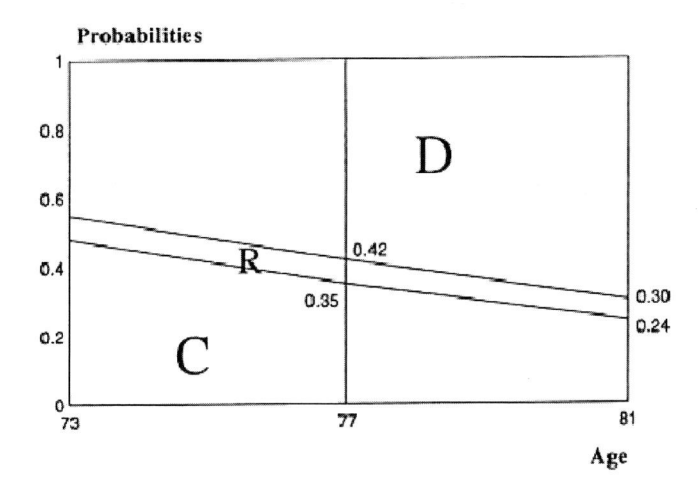

2.4(b) multinomial probability of survival of a male individual given observed age, from Table 2.6.
Figure 2.4. Diagrammatical representation of the multinomial response probability distribution given observed age.

There is strong evidence to suggest that poor health is related to non-survival in the community. It can be seen (Table 2.6) that the likelihood of non-survival in the community increases as (self-assessed) state of health declines. This is reflected in its negative parameter estimates (e.g. -0.76 for 'all right for age' and -1.31 for 'fair/poor' in Table 2.6).

Self-assessed state of health appears to influence the outcome probability in the sense that poorer health appears to accelerate leaving the community. This is again illustrated in Figures 2.5 (a) and (b). It can be seen that, over the period 1979-87 (Table 2.6) those 73 year olds (who were 65 in 1979) who in 1979 assessed their health to be 'fair/poor' are 2.4 times less likely to remain in the community and 1.7 times more likely to have died by 1987 than other 73 year olds who claimed to be in a 'good' state of health. Elderly individuals enter into residential care for several reasons, e.g. loneliness [56, 57]. Some studies suggest residential care causes loneliness whilst Dykstra and colleagues [56] suggested that entering residential care does not reduce loneliness. Deterioration of health in old age prompts more contacts, care and visits from close relatives, friends and neighbours [58]. This may, at least in part, explain why those in poor health have a lower probability of entry into residential care. Therefore, as shown in Figure 2.5(a), elderly individuals with a low probability of remaining in the community, possibly due to poor health, will have a high probability of dying, thus a low probability of entry into care. On the other hand, Figure 2.5(b) suggests that those elderly in good health appear to have a higher probability of remaining in the community and a lower probability of death and a slightly higher probability of entry into residential care.

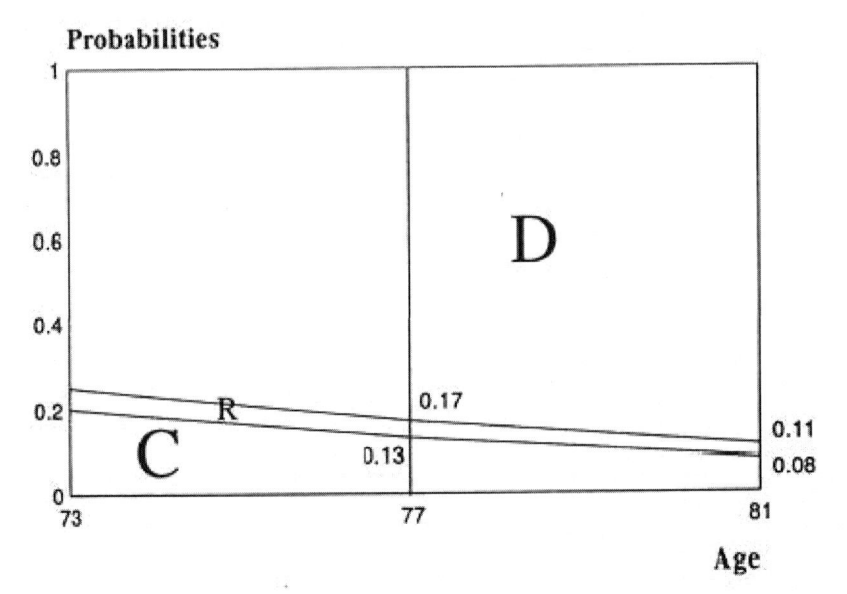

2.5(a) multinomial probability of survival for individuals in 'fair/poor' health for observed age, from Table 2.6.

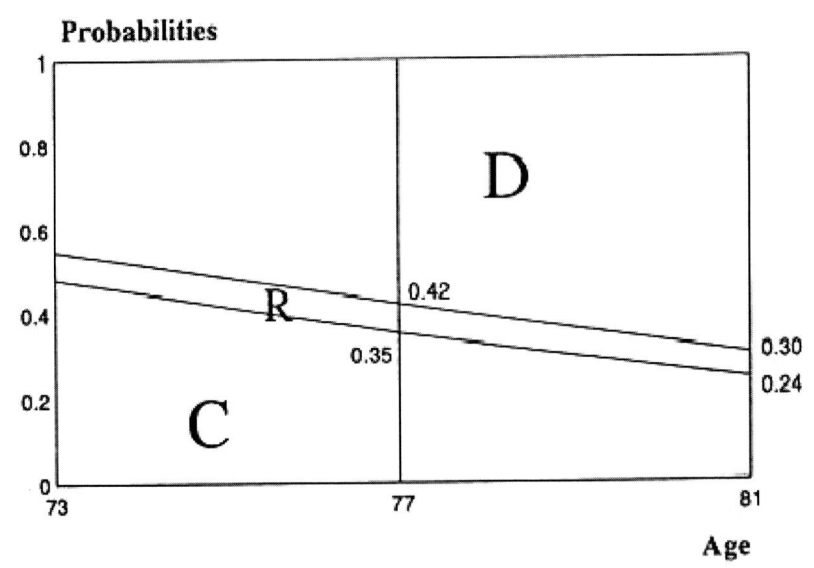

2.5(b) multinomial probability of survival for individuals in 'good' health for observed age, from table 2.6.

Figure 2.5. Diagrammatical representation of the multinomial response probability distribution given observed age.

The variable 'arrival age in community' appears to be positively linked with survival. There is strong evidence to support its inclusion in the model for the period 1979-87 (p=0.0013, Table 2.6). This suggests a long-term effect. Its positive parameter estimates suggest a positive influence, i.e. age of settling in the community appears to influence the probability of survival. Middle aged movers and retirement migrants (those who have moved more than 25 miles after the age of 60) have a greater chance of survival than retirement movers (those who move short distances after after the age of 60 - this group tends mainly to be locals). There is a degree of association between this variable, social class and network type [32]. The duration of staying in the community can reflect availability of kin; those who arrived in the community before or during child-rearing age are more likely to have a local kin network than those who arrived in middle or old age. Moreover, movement by those in the lower social class appears to take place mainly within the community. In this model, the variable 'arrival age in community', therefore, appears to control for the effects of both social class and network type.

2.5.5. Summary

This analysis suggests there is no direct relationship between survival and quality of life variables. To study the process of survival in the community fully, repeated observations on individuals are needed to define and measure varying degrees of dependency until death. For example, some individuals will enter into care for various reasons, possibly dependency, loneliness, or possibly for the reassurance of knowing that help is forthcoming in the face of increasing dependency. Do these groups have varying qualities of life and varying mortality rates? We need additional information such as time of entry into 'care', some measure of dependency, and data on the parameters measuring (or identifying) the process of entry into care.

To see how the multinomial model performs in comparison with the binomial logistic model fitted in Section 2.4, the results from the two models are reproduced in Table 2.7. Notice that for this table we have chosen to present parameter estimates (p.e.'s) along with their standard errors (s.e.'s) and associated p-values. This is the conventional way of presenting the results of fitting models but our main reason here is a comparison of the two models. Here we are not exploring how variables fit in a model but how models compare with each other. Although, ideally, both model should have had the same variables included to be able to compare p.e.'s and s.e.'s. Nevertheless, we are still able to compare the two models and use p.e.'s and s.e.'s as a guide.

In general, the p.e.'s are very similar but those of the multinomial model have much smaller s.e.'s. This may be evidence of a more powerful model because fuller use is made of the response data, but this difference may be due to the different sets of variables included.

The results for both models, in general, appear consistent. The multinomial model appears to agree with the binomial logistic model on the demographic variables 'age' and 'sex'. Furthermore, they also agree on the same measure for morbidity 'self-assessed health'. However, this variable appears to control fully for the effect of ill-health, the resulting dependency and impending death, i.e. the multinomial model excludes the variable 'visits from district nurse'. Similarly, 'arrival age in the community' appears to control fully for any social class effect and/or availability of a support network by excluding ethnicity. Therefore, over and above the well understood effects of age and sex, survival in old age may be governed by health status, level of dependency and availability of support networks (either informal or formal). However, the multinomial model allows a more effective use of additional information and enables exploration of outcome probabilities, not only of survival but also of survival in the community and of survival in care (see Figures 2.3-2.5).

Table 2.7. Comparison of the binomial and multinomial models fitted to the NWEP survival data

Variables	Binomial model (Survivor/deceased in 1987)			Multinomial model (in the community/in care/deceased)		
	p.e.	s.e.	p	p.e.	s.e.	p
Age	-0.11	0.02	(«0.00001)	-0.13	0.009	(«0.00001)
Sex			(0.00005)			(0.0001)
Male	0.00			0.00		
Female	0.85	0.21		0.76	0.12	
Health			(0.0001)			(<0.00001)
Good/excellent	0.00			0.00		
Alright	-0.72	0.23		-0.76	0.13	
Fair/poor	-0.124	0.27		-1.33	0.15	
Arrival age			(0.004)			(0.0013)
Long term	0.00			0.00		
Middle aged mover	0.86	0.28		0.80	0.15	
Retirement mover	0.16	0.33		0.19	0.18	
Retirement migrant	0.89	0.33		0.80	0.15	
District nurse visit			(0.025)			
No	0.00			-	-	
Yes	-0.62	0.28		-	-	
Ethnicity			(0.05)			
English	0.00			-	-	
Welsh	0.35	0.30		-	-	
½ Welsh	0.02	0.52		-	-	
British	1.65	0.62		-	-	
Other	0.54	0.71		-	-	

2.6. STATISTICAL MODELLING OF DURATION DEPENDENCE: SURVIVAL IN OLD AGE

The binary and multinomial models that were employed to analyse survival data in the previous two sections use only partial information i.e. only status at endpoint. An individual whose status in 1987 was recorded as deceased could have died at any point in time during the study window 1979-87. The individual may have died just after the 1979 interview or may have died just before the 1987 interviews; these are two very different outcomes. This level of information is lost in the logistic regression models presented in the previous sections.

A common problem is that it will take a very long time to observe all individuals until they die. In practice, the maximum 'duration' is taken to be the duration of the study window; in this case, 1979-87 for the NWEP. The structure of the survival data is shown in Figure 2.6. All individuals are observed either until death or to the end of the project. Those individuals who survive to the end of the project are called right censored individuals. Such right censoring does not, in general, prejudice modelling of survival durations.

The NWEP was designed primarily to explore how elderly people live in rural areas. As such, the main interests related to the elderly people's social networks, sources of care and support, well being and physical health, involvement in the community and access to amenities. The tracing of all 1979 respondents in 1983 and 1987 provided an outcome status originally so that individuals could be recruited to the second and third phase of the project. The project statistician was only appointed in the third phase of the project in 1987 when an effort was made, as part of the third phase, to collect dates of death. However, the interesting point here is the comparison of different models and of the different levels of insight gained.

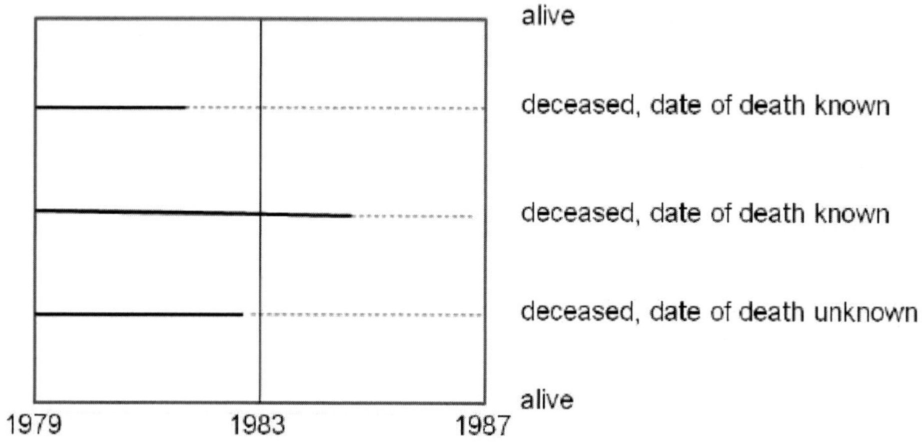

Figure 2.6. Diagrammatical representation of 'duration dependence' where the probability of survival is influenced by length of time survived.

2.6.1. Statistical Modelling of Survival Times

Here, survival time refers to the actual length of time an individual survived. Since all individuals were alive and in the community at the start of the project, the maximum survival time is equal to the length of the 1979-87 study 'window' with October 1987 being the cut-off point i.e. 8.5 years. The data are right censored. This means that all the individuals who were alive by the cut-off point will be assigned the maximum survival time of 8.5 years. Therefore, all sample members will have an observed duration (T). This type of data can be modelled routinely as described in Appendix IV.

2.6.2. Problem 1: Missing Durations

As mentioned at the start of this section, dates of death were collected retrospectively within a tightly specified period of time. The 1987 follow-ups revealed that 264 individuals had died over the eight year period up to October 1987 and dates of death were available for 224 cases. With the resources available, it had not been possible to trace the date of death for the remaining 40 cases. This complicated the modeling, which otherwise would have been a routine analysis using standard statistical packages.

The problem is that we could not afford to exclude the information from the 40 cases who had died but with unknown duration. If we had excluded these cases then we could have carried out the analysis routinely. We would not have known the extent to which the exclusion of these 40 cases would have introduced bias into the analysis. On the other hand, we will not know what effect the exclusion of 40 cases may have on the results. More information could only improve the analysis. Therefore, our problem was how to deal with this non-routine issue.

One way of dealing with such a situation is to think of three groups in the data: those individuals who were still alive in 1987, those who had died before 1987 and for whom date of death was known, and those who had died before 1987 with unknown date of death. The inclusion of the latter group makes the analysis non-routine and involves a purposely written computer program to handle this additional group.

2.6.3. Problem 2: A Substantive Issue

Social circumstances will have an impact on survival, in part, by affecting health and, possibly, dependency. Controlling for these variables may therefore result in an over-conservative, attenuated estimate of the effects of social circumstances. Reverse causality is also possible, with health and dependency influencing social circumstances. Excluding these factors may therefore exaggerate the effects of social circumstances. As emphasised in the introduction, we cannot unravel completely the complex causal relationships that are likely to exist between social circumstances, health, dependency and survival. We therefore adopted a pragmatic approach to this problem, repeating each analysis with and without the health and dependency variables.

2.6.4. Operationalisation of the Model with Missing Durations

It can be envisaged that there are three groups of individuals. Some were alive in 1987; let T_i be the duration of observation (8.5 years) for individual i in this group. Some died before 1987 at a known date; let T_j be the duration from 1979 to the date of death of individual j in this group. Finally, some died before 1987 at an unknown date; let T_k be the maximum possible survival duration (8.5 years) for individual k in this group. Then the likelihood contributions for individuals in each of the three groups are given by

$L_i = S(T_i)$,
$L_j = f(T_j)$, and
$L_k = 1 - S(T_k)$,

where f denotes the probability density of death and S the probability of survival. The first and second terms are standard for survival data subject to right censoring [59-61]; the third term has been included because of the missing dates of deaths.

A probability distribution for survival can be specified by its density, survivor or hazard function. In practice, it is often more convenient and useful to specify the probability distribution by its hazard, facilitating model formulation and model interpretation. A detailed account and discussion on survival analysis can be found in statistical text books, notably [24, 59-61]. A conventional log-linear specification was used (see Appendix IV) for the explanatory variables with $\lambda = \exp(\beta_0 + \beta_1 x_1 + \beta_2 x_2 + ...)$ where the $\{\beta\}$ are parameters to be estimated. It is noted that this may be written as a series of multiplicative terms, $\lambda = \exp(\beta_0)\exp(\beta_1 x_1)\exp(\beta_2 x_2)...$, aiding the interpretation of the effects of categorical variables. For example, the multiplicative effect q for an individual in category k of self-assessed health is calculated as:

$$q = \exp(\beta_{\text{health},k})$$

For an individual with poor health (β=0.87, from Table 2.10) q is calculated to be 2.4. Thus, individuals in this health category are estimated as having nearly 2½ times the death rate of individuals with the same characteristics but in excellent/good health (the reference group for self-assessed health).

For model fitting, an appropriate FORTRAN program was developed. The program incorporated NAG [62] optimization and matrix algebra subroutines to calculate the maximum likelihood function. In addition to the parameter estimates and standard errors, the program also produced the log-likelihood, likelihood ratio test statistic (χ^2) and its associated p-value. This program was further automated to carry out a variable selection process on the basis of the likelihood ratio test statistic (χ^2), see [28].

2.6.5. Variable Selection Process

In the previous sections, we discussed the reasons for adopting a 'forward substitution' model fitting procedure. Briefly, as shown in Table 2.8, variables were entered in the model one at a time with the 'best' additional variable added to the model at each stage. The improvement in the model as a result of adding each variable in turn was assessed by a likelihood ratio test statistic and the process ceased when no additional variable was significant at the 5% level.

At stage 1 (Table 2.8) all 30 explanatory variables were entered individually into the model and 18 were significantly related to survival at the 5% level. The significant factors came from all categories: demographic, socio-economic, social, quality of life, dependency and health. However, the social class variable was not significant, even at the 10% level. In so far as each explanatory variable was considered separately at stage 1 and its relationship with survival assessed, the analyses are comparable to those of Table 2.1 (Section 2.2). The results are reassuringly similar but not identical because the hazard model formulation utilizes the full information available on date of death, not just whether or not individuals survived to 1987.

Age emerged as the most important single variable at stage 1 and was added to the model. Controlling for age has a marked effect on the social variables; none remained significant at the 5% level. The social variables, including network type which was significant at the 1% level on its own, had been expected to be associated with survival.

The dominant effect of age is also revealed by the substantial reductions in the significance of the other previously significant variables. The only exception, gender, is readily understood. Women in the sample are, on average, older than the men because of their greater longevity. This age difference results in a rather higher mortality rate amongst the women than would otherwise be the case. The lower mortality rate for women due to the gender effect is, therefore, less marked when there is no control for age. These results for age illustrate how multicollinearity seriously undermines any attempt to interpret the bivariate relationships with survival. Age does not, in general, have high levels of association with the other variables; Table 2.2 shows that only one Cramer's υ exceeds 0.25. Nevertheless the associations are sufficient to induce misleading relationships between many of the other variables and survival.

The self-assessed health variable was the clear 'winner' at stage 2 of the model fitting procedure and this left three further variables significant at the 5% level: gender, home tenure (i.e. owner-occupier, tenant, etc.) and district nurse (i.e. attendance presages death). Each of these variables remained significant through the final stages. Indeed, it is notable that only one variable, which was significant at the 5% level failed to be included in the final model after controlling for age. This was the 'home help' variable which appeared to owe its significance to association with age and health. The final model is shown in Table 2.9.

The substantive issue of Sub-section 2.5.3 is tackled by repeating the model fitting without the health and dependency variables. No additional social variables were included in the model. The results are shown in Table 2.9; the values in parentheses are the results when the health and dependency variables were excluded from the model. It can be seen that the changes in the parameter estimates for the remaining variables were modest. The health variable and dependency measures do not appear to be important control variables in when examining the relationship between social characteristics and survival.

Table 2.8. An example of variable selection process

Variables	d.f	Stage 1	Stage 2	Stage 3	Stage 4	Stage 5
Demographic Variables						
Age	1	58.4***	included	included	included	included
Gender	1	3.9*	10.0**	13.6**	included	included
Household composition	2	6.3*	0.5	-	-	-
Marital status	2	6.8*	0.4	-	-	-
Number of children	1	2.1	-	-	-	-
Arrival age	3	1.6	-	-	-	-
Ethnicity	4	12.4*	8.6	-	-	-
Socio-economic Variables						
Income	2	11.1**	2.7	-	-	-
Social class	2	3.7	-	-	-	-
Home tenure	2	13.4*	10.1**	7.5*	7.7*	included
Social Variables						
Relative seen most	3	4.4	-	-	-	-
Frequency of contact with family	3	3.7	-	-	-	-
Number in network	3	7.5	-	-	-	-
Network type	4	16.7**	6.0	-	-	-
Hours spent alone	1	1.3	-	-	-	-
Quality-of-life Variables						
Isolation measure	1	4.1*	0.3	-	-	-
Loneliness measure	1	8.2**	3.6	-	-	-
Morale	2	9.2**	4.5	-	-	-
Self-assessed loneliness	1	3.6	-	-	-	-
Worry over bills	2	0.9	-	-	-	-
Health and Dependency Variables						
Self-assessed health	3	34.5***	21.5***	included	included	included
Health limited activities	1	12.2***	3.5	-	-	-
Doctor	1	10.4**	2.1	-	-	-
District nurse	1	17.5***	7.2**	3.9*	4.5*	5.4*
Home help	1	11.7***	4.6*	1.2	-	-
Private home help	1	4.2*	1.8	-	-	-

Hazard of death with Weibull specification; N=524; Likelihood ratio test statistic χ^2 and level of significance: *5%; **1%; ***0.1%.

2.6.6. Interpretation

It is clear that the elderly people's subjective assessment of their own health has high predictive value for subsequent survival. The inclusion of the 'district nurse' variable in the main model warns us that this subjective assessment is not a fully effective measure of ill-health, dependency and other aspects of frailty. However, self-assessed health is decidedly superior to the other indicator variables considered. From Table 2.9, the elderly assessing their health as 'all right for age' have about 1.5 times the death rate of those with excellent/good health. The figures for fair and poor self-assessed health are about 2 times and 2.4 times respectively. These results can be seen more clearly diagrammatically, by plotting the hazard rate for given values of the explanatory variable over time. For example, Figure 2.7 illustrates how the risk of dying over time varies from one category of (self-assesed) health to another. The hazard rate rises more steeply for elderly individuals who assessed their own health as poor than for those who assessed their health as good/excellent (other characteristics being the same: aged 65, male, owner occupier, who do not receive visits from a district nurse). It can be seen that the hazard rate for those in good/excellent health is much flatter than the hazard rates for those in other categories of self-assessed health, which rise more sharply and maintain an upward trend over time.

Table 2.9. Model fitting results controlling for duration dependence, N=524

Explanatory Variables (1979)	Parameter Estimates	Multiplicative Effect on the Hazard	χ^2	d.f	p
Gamma γ	1.4				
Age	0.61 (0.70)		41.5	1	«0.0001
Sex			14.8	1	0.0001
Male	0.00 (0.00)	1.00 (1.00)			
Female	-0.51 (-0.43)	0.60 (0.65)			
Home Tenure			8.5	2	0.014
Owned/mortgaged	0.00 (0.00)	1.00 (1.00)			
Rent	0.29 (0.40)	1.34 (1.49)			
Other	0.42 (0.42)	1.52 (1.52)			
Health			18.2	3	0.0004
Excellent/good	0.00	1.00			
All right for age	0.43	1.54			
Fair	0.67	1.95			
Poor	0.87	2.39			
District Nurse			5.4	1	0.0206
No	0.00	1.00			
Yes	0.37	1.45			
Log-likelihood	-743.4 (-756.98)				

Note: Values in parentheses are the results obtained when health and dependency variables were excluded from the analysis.

The socio-economic variable 'home tenure' appears to be related to mortality in old age. From Table 2.9, the elderly in rented accommodation have about 1.3 times, and those in the 'other' category (including living with relatives other than spouses) have about 1.5 times the death rate of owner occupiers, other factors being equal. It is noted that these figures may include some element of dependency over and above that represented by the other variables in the model. For example, those living with relatives may tend to be more frail. Nevertheless, the significance of the 'home tenure' variable suggests that survival is affected by socio-economic factors which are not adequately represented by the social class and income variables.

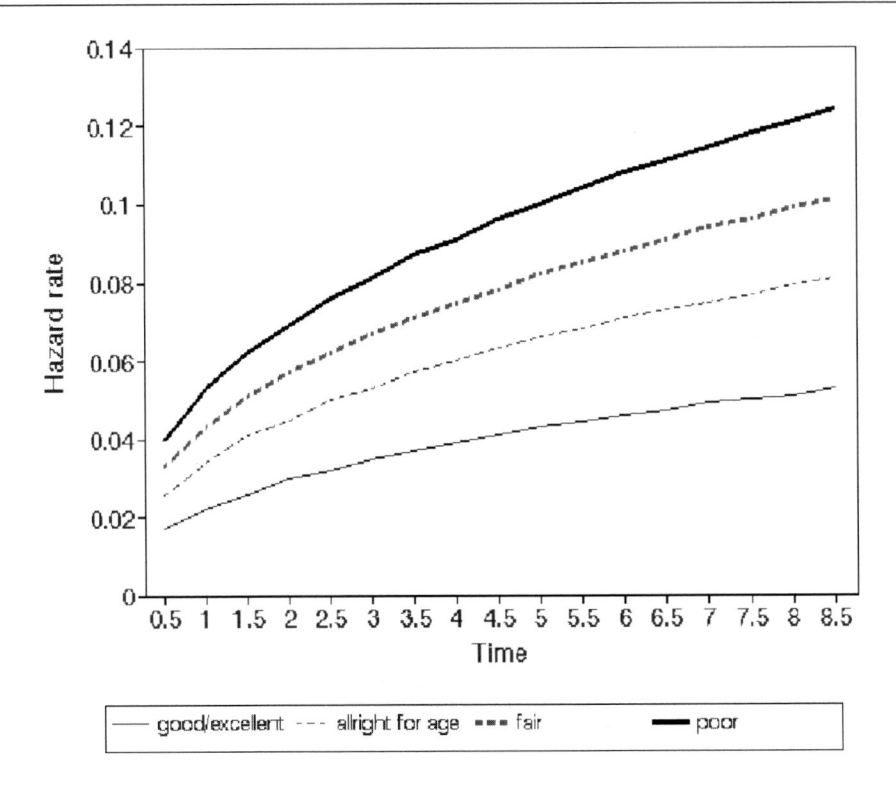

Figure 2.7. Diagrammatical illustration of how hazard rates vary by (self-assessed) health.

2.7. SUMMARY

To examine how the different models of survival performed we summarise the results for the three models in Table 2.10. Generally, the results from the binomial, multinomial and hazard models appear consistent. In particular, none of the results suggests any quality of life effect on survival, even when excluding the health and dependency variables from the model. The subjective assessment of dependency as measured by the variable 'state of health' appears to be a better predictor of survival than any other objective measures of dependency that were included in the analysis.

The multinomial model appears to agree with the hazard and binomial logistic models on the demographic variables age and sex. Furthermore, they also agree on the same measure for morbidity 'self-assessed health'. This variable appears to control fully for the effect of ill-health in the multinomial model i.e. it excludes the variable 'visits from district nurse'. The models differ, however, in the choice of socio-economic variables. The binomial logistic model includes two socio-economic measures: 'arrival age in community' and 'ethnicity'. The hazard and multinomial models each include one socio-economic measure: 'home tenure' and 'arrival age in community' respectively. Finally, it is emphasised that, with hazard modelling, we also obtain information about how mortality varies over time. This is illustrated by Figure 2.7.

2.8. CONCLUSIONS

With the cross-sectional modelling of survival, the multicollinearity issue was addressed. It was demonstrated that tackling this issue will help to reduce the number of explanatory variables thought to contribute to an outcome (survival in this case) to a manageable number. To some extent, accounting for multicollinearity also helped to explore and distinguish systematic effects in the data from random variations which tend to obscure any pattern. Advancing the analysis, from a standard logistic model to modelling multinomial response and duration survived, allowed us to take into account more information on individuals.

It is reasonable to assume that, when more information is included in the analysis, we may expect more informative results. However, this additional insight may be gained at a cost i.e. through increasing complexities in the model.

Table 2.10. Comparison of the three models fitted to the survival data

Explanatory Variables	Binomial model p.e.	s.e.	p	Multinomial model p.e.	s.e.	p	Hazard model p.e.	s.e.	p
Age	0.11	0.02	0.0000	0.13	0.009	0.0000	0.61	0.09	0.0001
Sex			0.0000			0.0001			0.0001
Male	0.00			0.00			0.00		
Female	-0.85	0.21		-0.76	0.12		-0.51	0.12	
Health			0.0000			0.0001			0.0004
Good/excellent	0.00			0.00			0.00		
Allright	0.72	0.23		0.76	0.13		0.43	0.14	
Fair/poor	1.24	0.27		1.33	0.15		0.70	0.16	
Arrival age in community			0.0040			0.0013			-
Long term	0.00			0.00			-	-	
Middle aged mover	-0.86	0.28		-0.80	0.15		-	-	
Retirement mover	-0.16	0.33		-0.19	0.18		-	-	
Retirement migrant	-0.89	0.33		-0.80	0.15		-	-	
District nurse			0.0250			-			0.0206
No	0.00			-	-		0.00		
Yes	0.62	0.28		-	-		0.38	0.15	
Ethnicity			0.0500			-			-
English	0.00			-	-		-	-	
Welsh	-0.35	0.30		-	-		-	-	
Half Welsh	-0.20	0.52		-	-		-	-	
British	-1.65	0.62		-	-		-	-	
Other	-0.54	0.71		-	-		-	-	
Home tenure			-			-			0.0140
Owner	-	-		-	-		0.00		
Rent	-	-		-	-		0.30	0.15	
Other	-	-		-	-		0.42	0.15	

Note: The signs of p.e.'s in the binomial and multinomial models have been reversed to be consistent with those of the hazard model, i.e. positive estimates now suggest increasing hazard.

The results for each model were discussed in the appropriate sections. Briefly, it is clear that **the 'district nurse' effect represents impending death** and thus health and dependency. To some extent, **the 'arrival age in community' effect also represents health and dependency**; those who moved to the area early in life are more likely to have established social and care networks. On the other hand, **the 'arrival age in community' effect is also a proxy for social class and income**, as is 'ethnicity'. Including additional information in the analysis, such as an extra category to distinguish between survivors in the community and survivors in care, appears to remove the dependency and social class effects represented by 'district nurse' and 'ethnicity' respectively. This additional information meant that the binomial model was no longer appropriate. Thus a slightly more complex multinomial model is more appropriate to take account of the new information. Similarly, analyzing the duration survived meant that we are dealing with a continuous response rather than a discrete outcome and thus the family of logistic models was not appropriate. So hazard models were applied. The results from this analysis suggest that the health and dependency variables directly influence survival over and above age and sex effect. However, the presence of 'district nurse' and to some extent 'home tenure' appear to 'mop up' some of the variation in survival rates due to frailty but had been left unexplained by the self-assessment variable. On the other hand, 'home tenure' may be a proxy for social class and socio-economic effects. However, the data suggest that those elderly people living in alternative accommodation, in particular with others, are more likely to be more dependent and less mobile.

As mentioned in Appendix IV, the Gompertz model was also fitted to the survival data. It was found to give very similar results for the explanatory variables but with a rather worse fit to the data (i.e. the log-likelihood was lower).

In summary, the appropriate method of analysis is dependent on the type and nature of the response subject to relevant substantive issues. For example, when variables are collapsed into fewer categories we may inadvertently place dissimilar individuals into the same category. However, one has to be aware that (substantively viewed) this may not be as important an issue analytically. For instance, if we are primarily interested in the number of deceased then it may be reasonable to categorise all the deceased individuals into one category. When the interest lies in exploring the factors that may influence survival, then individuals who died at the start of the project window may well be different to those who died at the end of this period (in this example a difference in duration of 8.5 years). When grouped together, it is not possible to utilize fully the explanatory power of explanatory variables such as health and dependency. To some extent, we have got around the problem through collecting additional information e.g. for the survival example, we collected more data on the length of time an individual survived. Dates of death were collected retrospectively and duration of survival was determined from the beginning of the project window until death [33]. The increased explanatory power in the statistical model we adopted comes from being able to account for each respondent's contribution.

We were not able to use the dynamics of explanatory variables in these models, e.g. the true effects of 'home tenure' as an indicator of socio-economic effect or dependency, or change in health status from 1979 to 1983 and to 1987. These issues will be discussed in Chapters 3 and 5.

Chapter 3

STATISTICAL MODELLING OF MORALE IN OLD AGE

3.1. INTRODUCTION

As discussed in Chapter 1, assuming that a survey study is designed and carried out appropriately, we will still have to deal with important issues of multicollinearity and omitted data; surveys do not collect data on all variables. Within a survey study, some variables are difficult to measure or cannot be observed (e.g. frailty, the feel good factor and personality) and thus are omitted from the study. When applying statistical models to data, these omitted variables are subsumed within the model's structural error term. Furthermore, surveys often collect subjective data (e.g perceptions and attitudes) as well as objective information (e.g. demographis), but in the analysis, the subjective variables are often treated as direct and independent effects. The subjective variables provide more than an objective measure for the variables being observed; they are often composite measures reflecting the overall mental and general state of the individual at the time of the survey. For example, in the old age survival study of the previous chapter, the variable 'self-assessed state of health' did not fully control for the health effect. In other words, other health and dependency variables such 'district nurse' were significant despite the presence of 'self-assessed health' in the model. Experience suggests that the elderly often under-report ill-health which they may associate with the process of ageing [33]. Thus, the variable 'self-assessed health' reflected more than the state of the individuals' physical health. It is, therefore, possible to envisage that the inclusion of subjective variables will lead to complex interactions with other included variables and with the error term. The main consequence of interactions with the error term is model mis-specification, leading to erroneous results and misleading conclusions.

One way of improving the study is to adopt a longitudinal design, to collect repeated observations capable of addressing the issues raised in Chapter 1. However, whilst longitudinal studies are becoming more common, most studies by local government, health sector and policy units are *ad hoc* and cross-sectional. For example, service satisfaction and attitudinal surveys, and surveys that collect information to inform policy formation lead to remain cross-sectional. So we may frequently find ourselves dealing with cross-sectional data. Although it is not possible to address the analytical issues related to the dynamics of human behaviour using cross-sectional data, we could explore the possibility of the existence of complex inter-relationships. This can be done simply by adopting a flexible and pragmatic approach to the statistical modelling approach (e.g. see [28, 29, 33, 63]) which involves taking full advantage of the richness of the data.

In this chapter, we investigate the issues raised in Chapter 1, namely multicollinearity, heterogeneity and omitted variables, and past behaviour. But first, we study how to anticipate the existence of the various sources of variation in the data and how to interpret results accordingly. We demonstrate these applications using morale in old age in this chapter and teenage smoking in Chapter 5.

3.2. MORALE IN OLD AGE: BACKGROUND

It is suggested that, given geriatric medicine's increasing focus on chronic disease, attention to morale is an important strategy for maximizing quality of life [64]. Sullivan [64] further suggested that improvement in the care of the elderly may be possible by getting physicians to detect and to treat problems with morale in old age. The literature reports a number of variables as correlates of morale in old age such as health, income, community activities, mobility and level of social support [20]. The relationship between morale in old age, depression and dementia is also well documented [65-68]. In practice, depression in old age is common, under-diagnosed and under-treated [69-73] and poor prognosis is associated with co-existing dementia and ill-health [68]. Depression in turn is related to reported health complaints [74], pain [75] and income [20]. Thus, there may be a true underlying relationship between morale and variables reported in the literature, however, there is a lack of clarity as to how these variables interact over time and whatever impact they have on morale. Indeed, in a series of papers, Ventegodt and colleagues [76-84] put forward a complex and sophisticated theoretical and philosophical framework for the scientific investigation of quality of life. They propose the construction of a global quality of life measure incorporating aspects such as perception and attitudes, well being, satisfaction with life, happiness, meaning of life, the biological information system, realizing life potential, fulfillment of needs, and objective factors. Most of these aspects are processes themselves and therefore are dynamic, with temporal dependencies within and between processes. For example, changes in morale may be due to mental and/or physical changes in individuals (e.g. increased frailty), or they may be due to constancy within individuals (e.g. personality); morale may return to its previous levels following an intervention or an event (e.g. bereavement).

One of the fundamental methodological problems, quite apart from the issues of defining and measuring quality of life, is disentangling the complex inter-relationships between quality of life and other variables. In reviewing the literature, Wenger [20] emphasized the difficulties inherent in attempting to disentangle the relationships of interest. As with any research based on survey data, it is difficult to distinguish systematic patterns from the random noise due to other variables. The flexibility of survey/observational studies to measure a wide range of subjective and objective variables adds complexities to analyses. Survey studies of elderly people living in the community do not often include measures of depression, morale or dementia all at the same time. In this context, in addition to the methodological issues of multicollinearity and the direction of causality, the issue of bias in the sample due to unmeasured or omitted variables also needs to be addressed. Wenger et al. [85] have addressed some of the difficulties associated with the analysis of survey data and reported an improved cross-sectional multivariate analysis to incorporate two fundamental issues of multicollinearity and the direction of causality. However, cross-sectional analyses do not allow an assessment of past behaviour (e.g. state dependence) and do not handle heterogeneity effects due to omitted variables (e.g. frailty).

Heterogeneity results when systematic but unmeasured characteristics of individuals contribute to responses over time. In survey studies, some individual characteristics are often omitted from the study because they are either unobserved or difficult to measure. Omitted characteristics, such as frailty, could lead to spurious relationships between the observed characteristics and the outcome variable. Past behaviour effects exist when the experience of a particular outcome itself changes the probability of experiencing that event on subsequent occasions. Again, it is clear that past behaviour cannot be addressed within cross-sectional designs. Heterogeneity and past behaviour effects are common when dealing with behavioural data and ignoring them will produce bias in deviance estimates and hypothesis tests [13, 14, 86].

Longitudinal studies provide an additional flexibility to increase control in the analysis; with panel data it is possible to control for heterogeneity and temporal dependencies, and to get a better understanding of the direction of causality [14, 87]. However, the traditional methods of analysing longitudinal data such as analysis of end points and analysis of variance do not fully utilise the properties of the data, and they exclude the heterogeneity effect [86, 88]. Multivariate methods such as factor analysis, cluster analysis and structural equations are aimed at reducing the dimensionality of a dataset and are available to improve cross-sectional studies. While these methods tend to reduce the number of variables to focus on, they can raise other complex questions about the nature of the process over time. Such outcomes are, in their own right, an important aspect of the results.

The North Wales Elderly Project (NWEP) project provides data on quality of life aspects such as morale, loneliness and self-assessed health. In this chapter, we explore the analysis of morale in old age. The main reason for selecting this topic is the interesting mix of challenges that we encountered during the analysis. First, we present a standard cross-sectional analysis followed by a modified cross-sectional analysis. We then explore alternative methods for the longitudinal analysis of morale in old age.

3.3. DATA

Wenger's [20] review of the literature suggests a number of social, socio-economic, demographic, health and dependency variables that may be influencing levels of morale in old age. In particular, better physical and mental health, social contact, friendship, activities and interaction and social support are suggested as being related to higher levels of morale.

The data used in the analyses come from the NWEP data bank. The structure of these data is shown in Figure 1.8 (Chapter 1, Section 1.5). The Philadelphia Geriatric Centre (PGC) morale scale [89] was administered as part of an extensive interview covering a wide range of topics. Unfortunately, the survey does not cover the duration an individual remained at a given level of morale. In the NWEP data set, morale and loneliness are available as recurrent measures making it possible to control for temporal 'state' dependence.

A measure of morale for each survey is available only for the old elderly survivors (see Figure 1.8). Cases with blank or missing values on their morale score sheet were dropped from the analysis, but the lowest score was allocated to those cases who found the scale rather upsetting. A total number of 38 cases of old elderly (aged 75+ in 1979) with a valid morale score were extracted from the dataset. A further limitation was the availability of the more objective health and dependency variables (Pfeiffer scales) only for 1983 and 1987. However, because of our interest in accounting for past behaviour in the analysis, we focus on analysing data from 1983 and 1987, with 1979 data providing information on previous levels of morale. This strategy also allows the inclusion of the Pfeiffer scales (objective measure of health) in the analysis. Two separate cross-sectional analyses were carried out. First, a cross-sectional analysis using the baseline data (1979) giving a sample of 507 cases with valid responses. Second, for the results in this chapter to be comparable with the results of fitting the longitudinal models reported in the next chapter, a cross-sectional analysis of the 38 survivors was carried out. However, the sample size can be increased by pooling the observations on these survivors from the 1983 and 1987 surveys to give a sample of 76 cases with valid morale measures.

As indicated above, a number of factors have been postulated as being related to morale: friends, confidants and social support; levels of activity or social participation; self-image and self-esteem; self-assessed health; loss; isolation. The appropriate variables in the NWEP data bank were extracted and a full list of explanatory variables used in this analysis is shown in Table 3.1 (also see Appendix I). The data include no appropriate variables related to activity or self-esteem. However, comparable variables for most correlates exist in the NWEP data set. Network types may be seen as life style measures. One of the characteristics of this variable is the nature of an individual's involvement in community activities (see Appendix I). Thus network type may stand as a proxy for community/social activity and participation. The Pfeiffer resource or dependency scales [90] (see also Appendix I) measure social resources, mental and physical health, activities of daily living and economic resources. These are interviewer assessments and thus are likely to be more objective measures than comparable self-assessed variables.

3.4. ANALYTICAL ISSUES

3.4.1. Continuous Response Variable

The distribution of morale for the baseline data (N=507) is highly skewed, as shown in Table 3.1. However, a Filliben test for normality showed a score of 0.94 and, on the basis of widespread application of this scale in the literature (e.g. [2, 91, 92]), the analysis proceeded without any transformation of the scale. The preliminary analysis here is confined to the testing of each variable on its own in a linear modelling framework (see round 1 in Table 3.2; for a fuller discussion see [85, 93]). It can be seen that there are ten variables which are not significant on their own. These factors include sex, marital status and number of years widowed.

Table 3.1. Distribution of morale for the baseline data (N=507)

Low morale	9%	(Aggregate morale score 1.0-2.0⁻)
Moderate morale	31%	(Aggregate morale score 2.0⁺-2.5⁻)
High morale	60%	(Aggregate morale score 2.5⁺-3.0⁻)

Table 3.2. Variable selection procedure: cross-sectional analysis of morale using the 1979 baseline data; N=507, p-values;* <=0.01, ** <=0.0001, *<=0.00001**

Explanatory variables	Round 1 p	Round 2 p	Round 3 p	Round 4 p	Round 5 p	Round 6 p	Round 7 p
Objective measures							
Sex	0.4	-	-	-	-	-	-
Age	0.04	0.76	-	-	-	-	-
Marital status	0.36	-	-	-	-	-	-
Number of years widow	0.48	-	-	-	-	-	-
Household composition	0.05	0.13	-	-	-	-	-
Has close relatives	0.78	-	-	-	-	-	-
Visits relatives	0.0003	0.32	-	-	-	-	-
Frequency see family	0.06	0.7	-	-	-	-	-
Relative seen most	0.45	-	-	-	-	-	-
Isolation measure	0.1	-	-	-	-	-	-
Network type	***	**	***	FIXED	FIXED	0.02	0.006
Who cares when ill	**	0.002	**	FIXED	FIXED	0.001	0.0002
Housebound	0.0009	0.27	-	-	-	-	-
Home tenure	0.06	0.03	0.02	FIXED	FIXED	0.51[1]	-
Have a phone	0.77	-	-	-	-	-	-
Hours spent alone	0.04	0.02	0.008	FIXED	FIXED	0.008	0.005
Nearest neighbour	0.27	-	-	-	-	-	-
Income	**	0.0003	**	FIXED	FIXED	**	**
Social class	0.11	-	-	-	-	-	-
Ethnicity	0.007	0.03	0.02	FIXED	FIXED	0.05	0.05
Subjective measures							
Presence of friends	0.0008			0.46	-	0.61[1]	-
People do favours	0.77			-	-	-	-
Self-assessed health	***			***	***	***	***
Health limited activities	***			**	**	***	***
Confidant	0.02			0.7	-	0.53[1]	-
Wish for more friends	0.0001			0.16	-	0.08[1]	-
R-squared			0.19		0.35		0.36

[1] Dropping these four variables at once makes little difference to the model.

3.4.2. Multicollinearity

As we have already established the importance of this issue in Chapters 1 and 2, we will not engage in a comparative study of univariate, bivariate and multivariate analyses of morale. Therefore, this issue will be addressed within the adopted statistical modelling framework in the same manner as in the previous chapter.

3.4.3. Past Behaviour

As mentioned before (see Chapter 1 and Section 3.2), past behaviour may have an impact on the current outcome. The only past behaviour variable that is available from the NWEP data set is morale in 1979 (as measured by the anglicised PGC morale scale) which may affect morale in 1983 (and in 1987). The data set does not offer duration or spells in any particular morale state. Nevertheless, this measure of morale will be exploited in the longitudinal modelling section (see Sub-section 3.8.2.2).

3.4.4. Omitted Variables

As mentioned in Chapter 1 and Section 3.2, omitted variables often relate to individual characteristics that have been left unmeasured (e.g. frailty) possibly because they are difficult to measure or are unmeasurable. Again, an advantage of longitudinal data modelling is the ability to address this issue whilst simultaneously controling for observed variables. This issue will be discussed in Section 3.8. Although we cannot formally address this issue within a cross-sectional analysis, using features of survey variables, we could adopt a pragmatic approach to gain insight into how reliable the results of our cross-sectional analysis may be. This is discussed in the next and cross-sectional analysis section (see Sub-section 3.6.2).

3.4.5. Subjectivity

A major problem with survey data is the inclusion of subjectively measured variables. Due to their possible relationship with omitted variables, subjective variables further complicate the issue of multicollinearity and could lead to overestimation of the statistical significance of such variables, thus leading to erroneous conclusions. In addition, because of the importance attached, in the literature, to the different roles of subjective and objective variables, we need to investigate the possible role that subjective variables play. We adopt the pragmatic approach of Chapter 2 to investigate these possible inter-relationships. In particular, three models are fitted and the results are compared. In the first model, the objective variables are assumed to control fully for the subjective effects (Figure 3.1 (i)) i.e. the model assumes that the subjective variables are intermediary effects. The second model assumes that subjective variables may be influencing morale independently over and above the objective variables (Figure 3.1 (ii)). The third model assumes that objective and subjective variables have independent and direct effects on morale (Figure 3.1 (iii)). The comparison of the results from these models could assist in interpreting the relationship between the subjective variables, the objective variables and the outcome, morale.

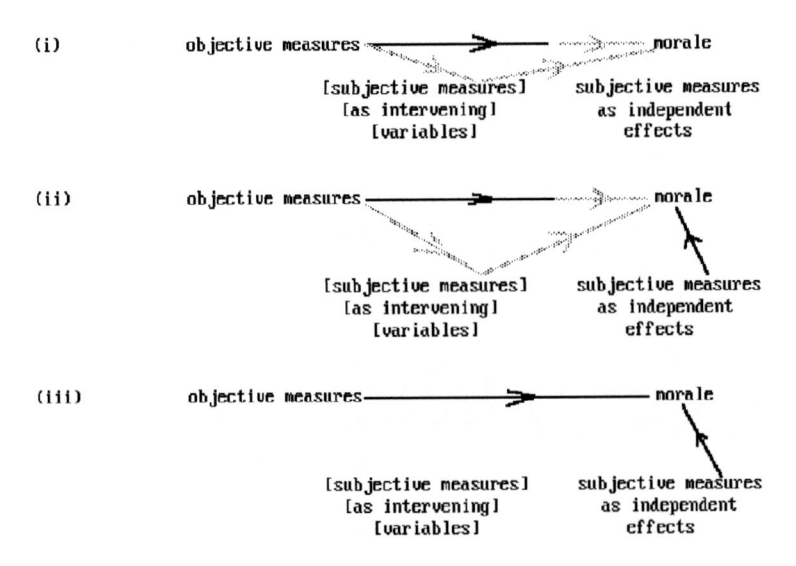

Figure 3.1. Modelling of morale: the pragmatic approach to improving control for omitted variables by distinguishing between subjective and objective variables.

3.5. STRATEGIES FOR ANALYSIS

We have longitudinal data on old elderly and we could proceed with the longitudinal modeling of morale in old age immediately. However, in the context of this book, and in general for comparison purposes, we propose to carry out a cross-sectional analysis as well as a longitudinal analysis of morale in old age. Simply having a longitudinal study design does not necessarily imply improved results without the application of appropriate longitudinal model(s). For example, Grundy [94, 95] applied a cross-sectional method to analyse data from a longitudinal study. As will be seen later, such applications will lead to model mis-specification, erroneous results and misleading conclusions.

One of the issues related to this data set is sample size. This limitation is, in part, due to the structure and the design of the project in 1979 (see [2]). There are only 38 cases of the old elderly for whom complete data across all 3 time points are available. We wish to account for past behaviour and utilise the objective health and dependency variables (Pfeiffer scores), so we are restricted to the 1983-87 data.

Therefore, the cross-sectional analysis may be carried out as two separate analyses: (a) analysis of the baseline data i.e. analysis of the 1979 data; (b) analysis of pooled data i.e. the 1983 and 1987 data pooled as one data set.

The first option gives a sample of 507 cases of elderly with a valid morale score. The second option produces a sample of 76 (2*38) cases with a valid morale score. For both cross-sectional analyses, the continuous aggregate morale score (taking values 1.0-3.0) is the response variable and the relationships between morale and various explanatory variables can be investigated using the normal regression model. For the variable selection and model fitting GLIM [52] was used.

A conventional regression model is assumed:

$$y_i = \beta_0 + \beta x_i + \varepsilon_i \qquad \varepsilon \sim N(0,\sigma^2)$$

the errors ε are assumed independent of the explanatory variables x. This assumption is relaxed in Section 3.8. The model selection is based on the F-ratio goodness of fit test statistic:

$$\frac{(RSS\ change)/(d.f\ change - v_1)}{(RSS\ of\ larger\ model)/(d.f\ of\ larger\ model - v_2)}$$

The associated p-values can be calculated using $\alpha\%$ level of significant and v_1 and v_2 degrees of freedom.

3.6. CROSS-SECTIONAL ANALYSIS OF BASELINE DATA

We follow the same process of variable selection that we used in Chapter 2. Once again this process is shown in Table 3.2. As discussed in previous chapters, the adopted statistical modelling framework allows us to account for multicollinearity using cross-sectional data. However, as pointed out in Section 3.3, there are a number of issues that cannot be addressed formally and directly when using cross-sectional data. Using a pragmatic method of formally distinguishing between objective and subjective variables, we could explore the relationship between morale and various explanatory variables, as shown in Figure 3.1.

3.6.1. Variable Selection Process

For the analysis of morale, for demonstration purposes, we present a mixture of forward iteration and backward elimination variable selection procedures. The values shown in Table 3.2 are p-values associated with the F-ratio test statistics, which represent the effects of explanatory variables on morale. The goodness of fit for the final models is based on the R^2 and is printed at the bottom of Table 3.2. Column 1 shows the p-values as a result of a bivariate fit within the same modelling framework, i.e. each variable is added to the null model (the model which only includes a constant) one at a time and its effect on the null model is noted. In Round 2 (column 2), the 11 variables which are significant at the 5% level are added to the model simultaneously. In Round 3 (column 3), variables are dropped out of the model one at a time (backward elimination) and their effect on the model is noted. This led to the elimination of five variables (age, household composition, visits relatives, frequency see family, and housebound) from the model all at once, which does not appear to affect the model significantly ($F_{11,49,0:0.05}=1.4$; p=0.16). Out of all the variables tested, only six variables remain significant, see column 3 of Table 3.2. final model 1 is as follows:

Model 1: objective measures only:- network type, who cares when ill, income, hours spent alone, home tenure, and ethnicity.

However, this model is a poor fit ($R^2=0.19$) explaining only 19% of the variation in data.

3.6.2. Testing for Subjectivity

We proceed to the next round of analysis which is testing the effects of subjective measures on morale over and above the objective measures. This is shown in Rounds 4 and 5, columns 4 and 5, of Table 3.2. Unlike the logistic regression presented in the previous chapter, we can, for a continuous response variable, fix the parameter estimates of the objective measures for the next model. This facility enables testing for subjective factors after allowing for the objective variables in the model. The parameter estimates of the objective variables are kept fixed and the subjective measures which were significant at the 5% level in Round 1 are then entered in the model (Round 4). In Round 5 (column 5), out of the five subjective variables entered in the model, the two health measures remain highly significant after backward elimination of confidant, presence of friend in the area, and availability of people to do favours. Final model 2 is as follows:

Model 2: fixed model 1 + self-assessed health, health limited activities.

It appears that the health measures have appreciable explanatory power over and above the objective measures. This model appears to be a better fit; R^2 has increased to 0.35

suggesting the additional effects of the subjective measures have improved the explanatory power of the model by 16%.

3.6.3. Unrestricted Model

The same modelling procedure is adopted in Rounds 6 and 7 (columns 6 and 7) of Table 3.2. Here, the effect of all the variables is tested without any restrictions and a model including both objective and subjective variables is selected. It can be seen that in this final round (column 7) only 'home tenure' drops out of the model while the two subjective measures remain in the model. Final model 3 is as follows:

Model 3: objective factors and subjective measures:-
network type, who cares when ill, income, hours spent alone, ethnicity;

self-assessed health, and health limited activities.

R^2 is increased to 0.36 and the explanatory power of the model is slightly improved by 1%. The model fitting results for the three models are shown in Table 3.3.

3.6.4. Interpretation of Table 3.3

In Model 3, the restrictions on the modelling process are lifted and the effects of the objective and subjective measures are tested within the same modelling process. Changes in the parameter estimates from Model 1 to Model 3, and from Model 2 to Model 3, provide some pragmatic indication of how the objective and subjective measures have distinct effects on morale. The results in Table 3.3 suggest very small increases in the parameters of the subjective measures from Model 2 to Model 3. This small change indicates that the subjective measures are predominantly related to morale as quite distinct effects over and above the effects of the objective measures. Conversely, the changes suggest that the subjective measures only have a very modest role as intervening variables between the objective measures and morale. However, this intermediary role may be sufficient to reduce the direct effect of some of the objective measures; most notably for 'network type' (although it remains highly significant there are appreciable reductions in the parameter estimates when subjective measures are included in the model) and 'home tenure' which ceases to be significant.

The variable 'home tenure' is classified as a socio-economic factor. It seems that, when controlling for health measures, the 'home tenure' link with morale is eliminated. This suggests that 'home tenure' may also be acting as a proxy for health. This is not surprising, as the link between health and socio-economic factors (e.g. social class, income, education, occupation, home tenure) has been documented (e.g. see [48]). Network type may also, in part, be acting as a proxy for health in model 1 and this provides an alternative explanation for the reduction in parameter estimates for this variable in model 3.

Table 3.3. Model fitting results of the cross-sectional analysis of morale using the 1979 baseline data, N=507, p-values: ** < 0.0001, * < 0.00001**

Explanatory variables	Models					
Objective measures	Model 1	p	Model 2	p	Model 3	p
Who cares when ill						
Spouse	0.00				0.00	
Relative	0.12	**	FIXED	-	0.09	0.0002
Friend/neighbours/others	0.03				0.01	
Missing - d/k	-0.41				-0.35	
Network type						
Family dependent	0.00				0.00	
Locally integrated	0.25	***	FIXED	-	0.13	0.006
Local self-contained	0.11				0.03	
Community focused	0.23				0.13	
Private restricted	0.02				-0.03	
Home tenure						
Owner occupier	0.00					
Local Authority rent	-0.14	0.02	FIXED	-	-	-
Private rent	0.002					
Other	-0.03					
Hours spent alone						
Up to 3 hours	0.00				0.00	
3-9 hours	-0.11	0.008	FIXED	-	-0.10	0.005
More than 9 hours	-0.16				-0.15	
Income						
Up to £39	0.00				0.00	
£40-79	-0.07	**	FIXED	-	-0.09	**
£80-99	0.05				0.005	
£100+	-0.28				-0.26	
Ethnicity						
Welsh	0.00	0.02	FIXED	-	0.00	0.5
Non-Welsh	0.11				0.08	
Subjective measures						
Self-assessed health						
Excellent/good			0.00		0.00	
Alright for age			-0.07	***	-0.09	***
Fair/poor			-0.31		-0.36	
Health limited activities						
Yes, limited			0.00	**	0.00	***
No, not limited			0.16		0.18	
R-squared	0.19		0.35		0.36	

3.7. POOLED CROSS-SECTIONAL ANALYSIS

The pooled cross-sectional model is a modification of the cross-sectional approach when data are available on the same individuals at different time intervals. The main justification for pooling the data is the increase in sample size and to include longitudinal information in the analysis. Even though the data will include observations on the same individuals at different points in time, the methodology is still cross-sectional.

For the pooled cross-sectional analysis, variables 'change in marital status' and the five Pfeiffer dependency measures (see Table 3.4, also Appendix I) are added to the variable list. The dependency measures (which are not available from the 1979 data set) are measures of social resources, mental health, physical health, capacity to perform activities of daily living and economic resources. The availability of (informal) help in case of illness (or emergencies) is a major contributory factor in assessing the score on the 'social rating' scale. For this reason, the variable 'who cares when ill' is dropped from the analysis. A cumulative Pfeiffer score [96] which sums dependency scores over the five scales as a continuous aggregate dependency measure is also included in the analysis.

A variable selection procedure similar to that of the previous analysis is used and is shown in Table 3.4. In Round 1, a bivariate analysis of morale within the modelling framework is conducted. Again, the values shown in Table 3.4 are p-values associated with the F-ratio test statistic, and the goodness of fit R^2 for each model is shown at the bottom of the table. At the next stage, all those objective variables, which were significant at the 10% level, were entered in the model, and then were excluded from the model one at a time. Note that, due to a much smaller sample size, the significance level was set at 10%. The backward elimination process proved unsuccessful; none appeared significant. This is another example of complex multicollinearity in data. When all the variables, which were significant on their own, are present in the model, the complex inter-relationships between variables make it impossible for the model to discriminate between them.

Forward variable selection was then employed and was more successful. On the basis of the result in Round 1 (column 1), Pfeiffer scale 3: physical dependence was selected as the 'best' variable to enter the model first (marked 'included' in column 2, Table 3.4). Then those variables which were significant at the 10% level in Round 1 were tested again one at a time and the results are shown in Round 2. The inclusion of Pfeiffer scale 3 in the model reduces the significance of other variables; some cease to be significant at the 10% level. The p-values for these effects are shown in brackets (Table 3.4; column 2; similarly for subsequent rounds in columns 3 to 7). As a result of this round, Pfeiffer scale 2: mental dependence is next allowed in the model. With this addition to the model, the remaining variables which were significant in Round 2 are no longer statistically significant. It must be noted that two other models were also fitted but are not shown in Table 3.4. The reason for fitting two other models is because, in Round 1, the p-values for two other variables: 'Pfeiffer 2: mental dependency' and 'cumulative Pfeiffer Score' are also small and close to the p-value of the variable 'Pfeiffer 3: physical dependency'. This means that any one of these variables could have been entered in the model first. Under such circumstances, it is advisable to investigate alternative models to ensure parsimony.

The first model to be examined was the one with the cumulative Pfeiffer score included first. This model appears to control for the variation in morale due to other variables (deviance or RSS=10.25, R^2=0.28) i.e. once cumulative Pfeiffer score is added to the model, all other variables become non-significant. The second alternative was the model with 'mental dependence' in first which results in a two-variable model: physical dependence, and mental dependence (deviance or RSS=9.84, R^2=0.31). This is the same model as the one shown in Table 3.4, i.e. the model with 'physical dependence' in first. On the basis of the smaller deviance and slightly better R^2, we proceed with the latter option. Final model 1 is as follows:

Model 1: objective measures only:- physical dependence (Pfeiffer scale 3), mental dependence (Pfeiffer scale 2).

Morale appears to be related to levels of dependency.

The parameter estimates of the above model are fixed in Rounds 4 and 5 to investigate the effects of the subjective measures on morale over and above the effects of the objective measures. Again, the forward substitution procedure is followed. Notice that, in Round 4, the effects of the subjective health measures, over and above the effects of the objective variables, are non-significant. This means that the more objective health measures (Pfeiffer 2 and 3) control fully for the subjective health variables. Therefore, in Round 5, only the variable 'confidant' is retained in the model (at the 10% level of significance). This suggests that, for the old elderly people, the additional subjective variables operate mainly through availability of a confidant. Final model 2 is as follows:

Model 2: Model 1 plus confidant.
R^2 is increased by 5% to 0.36.

As before, model 3 begins by relaxing the restrictions on model 1 (Rounds 6 and 7). In this case, the variable 'physical dependence' appears to be the clear 'winner' to enter the model first. Using the forward iterative procedure, the competition is between the subjective variable 'confidant' (p=0.003) and the objective Pfeiffer scale 'mental dependence' (p=0.02). It appears that, no matter which variable is entered in the model first, once 'confidant' is in the model, the variable 'mental dependence' ceases to be significant. Final model 3 is as follows:

Model 3: physical dependence (Pfeiffer scale 3), confidant.

There is a slight increase in R^2 of 1% to 0.37. The model fitting results are shown in Table 3.5.

3.7.1. Interpretation of Table 3.5

The results in Table 3.5 suggest a substantial increase in the parameter estimates for subjective measure 'confidant' from Model 2 to Model 3 which suggests that it operates as an intervening variable, partly reflecting mental dependence. This intermediary effect causes 'mental competence' to cease to be significant. It is not surprising that presence of a confidant acts as a buffer for the 'mental competence' effect. There appears to be a strong association between confidant and the variable 'Pfeiffer 2: mental dependence'. The Cramer's υ measures of association for confidant and all the Pfeiffer scores in 1983 and 1987 are shown in Table 3.6. It can be seen that confidant and mental health rating PF2 are highly correlated (υ=0.45 and υ=0.55; 1983 and 1987 respectively; Table 3.6). Out of the two, 'confidant' is the dominant effect which means that this variable controls for the variation in morale resulting from mental competence scores. It is also plausible that companionship in old age, as reflected by 'confidant', operates in the opposite direction to the effects from any lack of quality of life associated with lowered mental competence that may be affecting morale.

On the basis of this pooled cross-sectional analysis, the results of table 3.5 can be interpreted as follows:-

- The two objective explanatory variables (as measured by the Pfeiffer Scales) clearly suggest that greater physical and mental dependency may lead to lower levels of morale. On average, those highly dependent individuals, as shown by the physical dependency scale, score lower on the morale scale. Similarly, those high on the mental dependency rating scale also appeared to score lower on the morale scale. The results from the pooled cross-sectional analysis appear to suggest that dependency in advanced old age seems to explain at least 30% of the differentials in morale in old age, regardless of other objective socio-economic or subjective self-assessment measures of well-being.

- Having a confidant, or a perception thereof, appears to be positively correlated with morale; availability of a confidant increases levels of morale compared to not having a confidant. This variable appears to include any mental dependency effect measured by PF2 (Pfeiffer 2: mental dependency). Those who cited 'spouse' as their confidant appear to be more likely to score higher on the morale scale than those without a confidant.

Table 3.4. Variable selection procedure: pooled cross-sectional analysis of morale in 1983 and in 1987, N=76, p-values: based on F-ratio test statistic, significance @ 10%

Explanatory variables	Round 1 p	Round 2 p	Round 3 p	Round 4 p	Round 5 p	Round 6 p	Round 7 p
Objective measures							
Sex	0.65	-	-	-	-	-	-
Age	0.44	-	-	-	-	-	-
Marital status	0.62	-	-	-	-	-	-
Change in marital status	0.21	-	-	-	-	-	-
Number of years widowed	0.5	-	-	-	-	-	-
Household composition	0.68	-	-	-	-	-	-
Has close relatives	0.8	-	-	-	-	-	-
Visits relatives	0.02	(0.19)	-	-	-	-	-
Frequency see family	0.62	-	-	-	-	-	-
Relative seen most	0.5						
Isolation measure	0.14	-	-	-	-	-	-
Network type	0.03	(0.15)	-	-	-	-	-
Housebound	0.05	(0.5)	-	-	-	-	-
Home tenure	0.2	-	-	-	-	-	-
Have a phone	0.55	-	-	-	-	-	-
Hours spent alone	0.66	-	-	-	-	-	-
Nearest neighbour	0.95	-	-	-	-	-	-
Income	0.46	-	-	-	-	-	-
Social class	0.13	-	-	-	-	-	-
Ethnicity	0.19	-	-	-	-	-	-
Pfeiffer 1 (Social rating)	0.005	0.07	(0.53)	-	-	-	-
Pfeiffer 2 (Mental dependence)	**	0.02	included	FIXED	FIXED	0.02	(0.39)
Pfeiffer 3 (Physical dependence)	***	included	included	FIXED	FIXED	included	included
Pfeiffer 4 (Daily activities)	0.003	(0.97)	-	-	-	-	-
Pfeiffer 5 (Economic rating)	0.14	-	-	-	-	-	-
Cumulative Pfeiffer	***	0.023	(0.46)	-	-	-	-
Subjective measures							
Presence of friends	0.09			(0.21)	-	0.04	(0.41)
People do favours	0.3			-	-	-	-
Self-assessed health	0.002			(0.42)	-	(0.3)	-
Health limited activities	0.0006			(0.96)	-	(0.98)	-
Confidant	0.003			0.07	included	0.003	included
Wish had more friends	0.23			-	-	-	-
R-squared			0.31		0.36		0.37

Table 3.5. Model fitting results of the pooled cross-sectional analysis of morale in 1983 and in 1987, N=76 - ** < 0.0001, *** < 0.00001

Explanatory variables	Models					
Objective measures	Model 1	P	Model 2	p	Model 3	p
Pfeiffer Scale						
Mental dependence	-0.16	0.02	FIXED	-	-	-
Physical dependence	-0.14	0.002	FIXED	-	-0.18	***
Subjective measures						
Confidant						
No-one			0.00		0.00	
Spouse			0.35	0.07	0.54	0.003
Other			0.16		0.32	
R-squared	0.31		0.36		0.37	

Table 3.6. Cramer's υ measures of association between 'confidant' and the Pfeiffer scales

	PF1[#]		PF2[#]		PF3[#]		PF4[#]		PF5[#]		CMPF[*]	
Year	83	87	83	87	83	87	83	87	83	87	83	87
Confidant 83[+]	0.34	0.57	0.45	0.41	0.20	0.29	0.35	0.36	0.18	0.38	0.18	0.27
Confidant 87[+]	0.36	0.59	0.27	0.55	0.30	0.54	0.25	0.55	0.23	0.54	0.15	0.52

[#] Pfeiffer scores: PF1 ≡ social rating, PF2 ≡ mental health rating, PF3 ≡ physical health rating; PF4 ≡ daily activity rating, PF5 ≡ economic resources rating.
[*] aggregated cumulative Pfeiffer score
[+] Confidant ≡ no-one, spouse, other

3.8. LONGITUDINAL MODELLING OF MORALE IN OLD AGE

As discussed in the introduction and in previous chapters, a common problem in the analysis of cross-sectional studies is the implicit assumption that changes in explanatory variables will produce commensurate changes in morale. Apart from problems of control, as already emphasized in this book, this assumption may be untenable: because of temporal dependence, morale may depend not only upon social and other characteristics at a point in time, but also upon prior levels of morale. There may, for example, be inertial tendencies, with individuals slow to react to changes in circumstances. In other words, explanatory variables may change from one point in time to another but morale may not. For example, state of health of an individual may change from 'good' to 'allright for age' but morale levels may stay unchanged, whilst losing a confidant may adversely affect morale levels. But this effect may be temporary and morale could return to its previous level after a period of time.

Event history or longitudinal data are better suited to studies of social processes for two main reasons. First, we can obtain improved 'control' for the variables omitted from the analysis thereby reducing the risk of inferring cause and effect from a spurious relationship. Second, we can study the dynamics of change, e.g. whether levels of morale tend to persist over time. This section, therefore, seeks to investigate the association between explanatory variables and morale while controlling for temporal dependence and residual heterogeneity. The NWEP data bank contains repeated measures on morale, health and some other relevant explanatory variables.

Consider the NWEP data structure again (Figure 1.8): a number of individuals are observed, each up to three times over an eight-year period. For a given response vector (y_i) from this data set (e.g. morale in this case) for each individual or case we have:

observed response = {morale in 1979, morale in 1983, morale in 1987}

denoted by

$$y_i = \{y_{i1} \mid y_{i2} \mid y_{i3}\}$$

and for each y_i we have a vector of explanatory variables:

observed variables = {age, sex,... in 1979 | age, sex,... in 1983 | age, sex,... in 1987}

denoted by

$$x_i = \{x_{ij1} \mid x_{ij2} \mid x_{ij3}\}$$

where j=1,...,k refers to the number of relevant observed explanatory variables for each observed y. This data structure is a typical longitudinal structure where in general N cases or individuals are observed repeatedly up to T times:

$$y_i = \{y_{i1} \mid y_{i2} \mid ... \mid y_{iT}\}$$

and

$$x_i = \{x_{ij1} \mid x_{ij2} \mid ... \mid x_{ijT}\}$$

It can be seen that the y_i vector forms a cluster: the elderly individual i interviewed in years 1979, 1983 and 1987 forms cluster i. This means that individual i in the 1979 data set is the same individual as in the 1983 and 1987 data sets. In effect, individuals are used as their own controls and therefore, it will be inappropriate to treat the data as though they are generated from independent cases. The conventional regression model could not be applied to such a data structure.

Consider the conventional regression model:

$$y_i = \beta_0 + \beta x_i + \zeta_i \qquad (3.1)$$

where the ζ_i are independent and identically distributed (i.i.d.) error. An important feature of data that are structured in a hierarchy of clusters is that individuals in the same cluster will be more similar than those in different clusters. When applying equation (3.1) to hierarchical data, therefore it violates the zero correlation assumption, and as a consequence standard errors are underestimated. The solution to this problem is to adopt a 'variance component' specification with different error terms for each level of the hierarchy [12]. Applying a variance component specification to equation (3.1) gives:

$$y_{it} = \beta_0 + \beta \underline{x}_{it} + \theta_i + \varepsilon_{it} \qquad (3.2)$$

where ε is the i.i.d. random error, θ are the additional individual-specific error terms (often referred to as nuisance parameters), y_{it} is the response and $\underline{x}_{it}$ is the vector of explanatory variables for the ith individual at time t. Notice that the nuisance parameter (θ_i) is assumed to be time-constant.

3.8.1. Methods of Controlling for Time-Constant Residual Heterogeneity

It is not possible to estimate the nuisance parameters simultaneously with the structural parameters. It is therefore necessary to eliminate the error terms before model fitting. In practice, this can be achieved in two ways: a) by conditioning on a sufficient statistic (see Sub-sections 3.8.1.1 and 3.8.1.2), and b) by integrating the nuisance parameters out of the likelihood (see Sub-section 3.8.1.3). The latter is also known as the marginal likelihood method.

The conditional likelihood method uses only the within- or intra-individual variation for inference, while the integrated or marginal likelihood method uses both intra- and inter-individual variation for inference. Both methods seek to control for 'residual heterogeneity' but in different ways. Both methods distinguish between the two sources of variation: omitted heterogeneity through the random effects (θ_i) and through the i.i.d. errors (ε_{it}). Computationally, the problem is how to deal with the additional nuisance parameters (θ) and structural parameters (β) simultaneously.

The conditional likelihood method attempts this by conditioning on a sufficient statistic in such a way that change over time is detected. This will result in loss of information due to the exclusion of time-constant variables such as sex. The conditional likelihood method can therefore be restrictive as only one source of information, i.e. the time-variant variables, is used. The same problem, of how to deal with the nuisance parameters and the structural parameters simultaneously, exists for the integrated likelihood method. This method eliminates the nuisance variables by integrating them out of the likelihood hence it is often referred to as the integrated likelihood method.

3.8.1.1 Conditional Likelihood Method: Continuous Response Variable

This method controls for heterogeneity by conditioning the data on a sufficient statistic. First, we must eliminate θ from the equation so that the regression parameters of primary interest can be estimated using the available estimation techniques. Second, the method of conditioning the data on a sufficient statistic will depend on the nature of the response variable i.e. whether a response variable is continuous or categorical.

For a continuous response variable such as morale in old age, a sufficient statistic can be achieved simply by differencing the regression at times t and (t+1) [97, 98] as follows:

Consider equation (3.2) at time t:

$$y_{it} = \beta_0 + \beta x_{it} + \theta_i + \varepsilon_{it}$$

and the same equation for time (t+1):

$$y_{i(t+1)} = \beta_0 + \beta x_{i(t+1)} + \theta_i + \varepsilon_{i(t+1)}$$

then a sufficient statistic is $y_{i(t+1)} - y_{it}$:

$$y_{i(t+1)} - y_{it} = \beta(x_{i(t+1)} - x_{it}) + (\varepsilon_{i(t+1)} - \varepsilon_{it}) \qquad (3.3)$$

where t is the year 1979, (t+1) is the year 1983, θ_i's are the individual-specific random effects (heterogeneity) and ε_{it}'s are the i.i.d. errors. This method of conditioning the data leads to the elimination of the nuisance parameters θ from the model and all the constant terms including β_0. Model fitting may be carried out in any statistical package such as GLIM, LIMDEP, NLOGIT, R,SABRE, SAS, STATA. For this exercise we used the F-ratio goodness of fit test statistic as described in the cross-sectional analysis (Section 3.5).

When fitting such a model, care must be taken with the categorical explanatory variables. The categorical variables cannot be treated in the same manner as continuous variables. They must be recoded first as a set of dummies taking values (0,1). Any change at time (t+1) after subtraction should then show as '+/-1' and no change as '0'. The resulting dummy variables taking values (-1,0,1) could then be assumed to be discrete continuous covariates. Note that, during the model fitting process, each variable is represented by the set of dummy variables, i.e. when testing for the effect of a categorical variable, all the dummy variables representing that categorical variable must be entered in the model at the same time.

3.8.1.2. Conditional Likelihood Method: Binary Response Variable

Figure 3.2 shows how a change in a binary (0/1) response variable may be detected from one point in time to another. In other words, when adding two binary (0/1) variables, a value of one (1) represents change while a value of zero (0) or two (2) represents no change in that variable. With the conditional likelihood, method we are interested in cases whose status has changed over time, for whom a sufficient statistic is: $y_{t+1} + y_t = 1$ ([98], see Appendix VI).

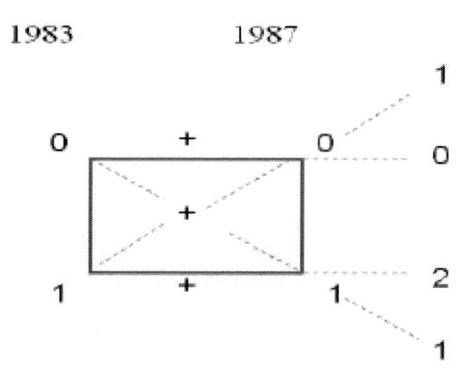

Figure 3.2. Possible status of a binary outcome over the interval 1983-87.

3.8.1.3. Marginal or Integrated Likelihood Method

This method of controlling for temporal dependence and residual heterogeneity is more advantageous because control is not restricted to time-variant factors. With this method, inference is based on both inter- and intra-individual variation, i.e. non-time-varying explanatory variables such as 'sex' could also be controlled for. Hence, all available information in the data set is utilised. However, the model is still restricted by the assumption of independence of the error terms θ and ε from the explanatory variables; the model assumes that these are not correlated with the included explanatory variables. Again, the two different types of response (e.g. categorical, continuous) require different treatments. For more details on ways of modelling a continuous response and a binary response using the marginal likelihood method, see Appendices VI and VII.

3.8.2. Longitudinal Analysis of Morale in Old Age

Here, as in the cross-sectional analysis (Section 3.6), morale in old age is treated as a continuous response variable, therefore both the conditional and integrated likelihood methods are appropriate ways of analysing the morale data. We demonstrate both methods.

Data from the NWEP data bank were extracted using the list of explanatory variables suggested in Section 3.6. There are two data limitation issues to address:

i. as shown in Figure 1.8, only the old elderly survivors (aged 75+ in 1979) have been surveyed at all three times (1979, 1983 and 1987);
ii. some variables of interest, e.g. the Pfeiffer scores, are only available at two times (1983 and 1987).

One approach would be to include all respondents from 1979: some will have one record of observation, some will have two records, and some will have three records (1979/1983/1987). However, a pragmatic approach is to concentrate on those old elderly cases who were surveyed in 1983. The disadvantage is the loss of data, but the advantage is that we can include the objective measures of health introduced in the 1983 survey. Furthermore, this approach will provide the 1979 data which will allow us to test the past behaviour effects, as will be seen later.

3.8.2.1. Conditional Likelihood Method

The model represented by equation (3.3) was adopted. Dummy variables representing the change in explanatory variables from 1983 to 1987 i.e. $(x_{i(t+1)}-x_{it})$ were created. Some of the explanatory variables were multi-categorical and differencing explanatory variables with more than two categories has no meaning. As mentioned earlier, to resolve this problem, categorical explanatory variables were converted into blocks of binary (0/1) variables. When differencing a binary categorical variable observed in 1983 and 1987, any change should then show as '+/-1' and no change as '0'. The resulting dummy variables taking values (-1,0,1) were then assumed to be discrete continuous covariates.

The variable selection process parallelled the one described in the cross-sectional analysis section (see Figure 3.1) and is summarized in Table 3.7. The results of the bivariate analyses in Round 1 (of stage 1, Table 3.7) show that there are only five objective variables which are significant at the 10% level. It is therefore reasonable to begin variable selection by fitting the full model. Explanatory variables are then dropped from the full model one at a time, their effect on the fitted model is noted and they are then put back in the full model. A number of variables was found to be non-significant. Dropping all non-significant variables from the full model has a significant effect (p=0.06), a clear case of multicollinearity. Backward elimination variable selection proceeded by excluding the least significant variable from the full model. The competition appears to be between 'cumulative Pfeiffer score' and 'has close relatives'.

Table 3.7. Variable selection process: conditional likelihood method, morale in 1983 and in 1987, N=38, p-values: based on F-ratio test statistic, significance @ 10% level

	Stage 1				Stage 2		Stage 3		
Explanatory variables	Round 1	Round 2	Round 3 Model 1	Round 4 Model 2	Round 5 Model 1	Round 6 Model 2	Round 7	Round 8	Round 9
	p	p	p	p	p	p	p	p	p
Objective measures									
Frequency see family	0.23	-	-	-	-	-	-	-	-
Relative seen most	0.32	-	-	-	-	-	-	-	-
Household composition	0.32	-	-	-	-	-	-	-	-
Has close relatives	0.05	0.1	0.034	-	FIXED	-	0.27	0.23	-
Isolation measure	0.44	-	-	-	-	-	-	-	-
Home tenure	0.88	-	-	-	-	-	-	-	-
Network type	0.17	-	-	-	-	-	-	-	-
Income	0.44	-	-	-	-	-	-	-	-
Bedfast	0.18	-	-	-	-	-	-	-	-
Number of years widow	0.37	-	-	-	-	-	-	-	-
Visit relatives	0.87	-	-	-	-	-	-	-	-
Age	0.89	-	-	-	-	-	-	-	-
Have a phone	0.32	-	-	-	-	-	-	-	-
Hours spent alone	0.01	0.01	0.01	0.01	FIXED	FIXED	0.09	0.01	0.01
Nearest neighbour	0.25	-	-	-	-	-	-	-	-
Pfeiffer Scales:									
Social rating scale	0.06	0.86*	-	-	-	-	-	-	-
Mental health rating	0.22	-	-	-	-	-	-	-	-
Physical health rating	0.17	-	-	-	-	-	-	-	-
Activities of daily living	0.17	-	-	-	-	-	-	-	-
Economic resources	0.20	-	-	-	-	-	-	-	-
Cumulative Pfeiffer score	0.045	0.34	-	0.06	-	FIXED	0.34	0.06	0.05
Marital status (m.s.)	0.51	-	-	-	-	-	-	-	-
Change in m.s.	0.76	-	-	-	-	-	-	-	-
Subjective measures									
Presence of friends	0.01				0.006	0.003	0.04	0.02	0.01
People do favours	0.65				-	-	-	-	-
Self-assessed health	0.015				0.13	0.05	0.16	0.15	0.05
Health limited activities	0.87				-	-	-	-	-
Confidant	0.13				0.25	0.42	0.4	-	-
Wish for more friends	0.3				-	-	-	-	-
R-squared			0.31	0.29	0.43	0.53			0.56

We adopt the pragmatic approach and fit two models: one with 'has close relatives', 'hours spent alone' and no other objective variables (R^2=0.31, Round 3), and the other with 'cumulative Pfeiffer score', 'hours spent alone' and no other objective variables (R^2=0.29, Round 4). The latter appears to be a slightly poorer fit.

In Rounds 5 and 6, the parameter estimates of these two models were fixed and the effect of the subjective measures was investigated. Model one, with its parameter estimates fixed, led to the inclusion of the variable 'presence of friend in the area' (with R^2=0.43, Round 5), while the second model improved with the inclusion of 'presence of friend in the area' and 'self-assessed health' (with $R^2=0.53$, Round 6).

In Round 7, variable selection continued by allowing variables, which were significant at the 10% level in Round 1, to enter the model. The least significant variable 'confidant' is dropped in Round 7 and then in round 8, 'has close relatives' is removed. The remaining variables all appeared to be significant at the 5% level. There is a slight improvement in the model $R^2=0.56$. At this stage (Round 7), two models were fitted. The first is the result of the variable selection process (including cumulative Pfeiffer score), and the second forced 'has close relatives' into the model in place of the cumulative Pfeiffer score and self-assessed health. The latter model gives, however, a poorer fit ($R^2=0.44$ compared to $R^2=0.56$). The final results are summarized in Tables 3.8a and 3.8b. The values in parentheses given in stage 3 of Table 3.8b are the results from the second model which includes 'has close relatives'.

The comparison of the parameter estimates resulting from the above model fitting provides some clues about the role of subjective effects as intervening or direct effect on morale. In Table 3.8a, there is a marginal increase in the parameter estimates of 'presence of friends' and 'self-assessed health' from Model 2 to Model 3. This small increase suggests that both these subjective measures are predominantly related to morale as quite distinct effects over and above the effects of the objective measures. Conversely, the change shows that the 'presence of friends' only has a modest role to play as an intervening variable between the objective measures and morale. However, this is sufficient to reduce slightly the direct effect of the objective variable 'hours spent alone'. Similarly, in Table 3.8b, the small increase in the parameter estimate of 'presence of friend in the area' seems to be sufficient to eliminate the objective variable 'has close relatives' from the model and leads to the inclusion of an additional objective variable 'cumulative Pfeiffer score' and a subjective variable 'self-assessed health'.

Table 3.8a. Model fitting results using conditional likelihood method, morale in 1983 and in 1987, N=38, significance at 10% level

Explanatory variables	Model 1					
Objective measures	Stage 1	p	Stage 2	p	Stage 3	p
Hours spent alone						
Up to 3 hours	0.15				0.04	
3-9 hours	-0.32	0.02	FIXED	-	-0.34	0.01
More than 9 hours	0.00				0.00	
Pfeiffer scale						
Cumulative score	-0.03	0.06	FIXED	-	-0.03	0.05
Subjective measures						
Presence of friends						
Yes			0.00	0.004	0.00	0.004
No			0.42		0.46	
Self-assessed health						
Excellent/good			-0.13		-0.17	
Alright for age			-0.24	0.05	-0.26	0.05
Fair/poor			0.00		0.00	
R-squared	0.29		0.53		0.56	

Table 3.8b. Model fitting results using conditional likelihood method, morale in 1983 and in 1987, N=38, significance at 10% level, 'close relatives' forced in

Explanatory variables	Model 2					
Objective measures	Stage 1	p	Stage 2	p	Stage 3[*]	p
Hours spent alone						
Up to 3 hours	0.15				(0.07)	
3-9 hours	-0.35	0.01	FIXED	-	(-0.38)	(0.003)
More than 9 hours	0.00				(0.00)	
Has close relatives						
Yes	0.00	0.03	FIXED	-	(0.00)	
No	-0.32				(-0.32)	(0.015)
Subjective measures						
Presence of friends						
Yes			0.00	0.006	(0.00)	
No			0.41		(0.43)	(0.004)
R-squared	0.31		0.43		(0.44)	

*The model fitting results at stage 3 are the same as those at stage 3 in table 3.8a. The values in parentheses are the results of model fitting excluding 'cumulative Pfeiffer score' and 'self-assessed health'. This model appears to be a poorer fit (R^2=0.44 compared to R^2=0.56 for model 1).

On the evidence provided by the application of the conditional likelihood method to the data on morale in old age, Table 3.8a and 3.8b can be interpreted as follows:-

- The cumulative Pfeiffer score appears to be marginally significant (p=0.05), although its effect on morale seems small. Higher scores on this scale suggest higher levels of dependency and vice versa. However, each Pfeiffer scale takes a value between 1 and 5. The cumulative score takes a value between 5 and 25 (see Appendix I). The result for this variable can be interpreted as follows: on average, an increase of one point on the cumulative dependency scale results in a reduction of 0.15 (0.03*5) points on the morale scale (other characteristics being the same).
- Those who claimed to spend up to 3 hours on their own appear to score about 0.04 points higher on the morale scale than those who said more than 9 hours (other characteristics being the same). The individuals scoring proportionally lowest on the morale scale (-0.34) appear to be those who said they had between 3 and 9 hours alone.
- The results for the variable 'presence of friends' in Tables 3.8a and 3.8b are contrary to intuition. Although it is highly significant (p=0.004), it appears that those who claimed there was no one in the area they could call a real friend, scored higher on the morale scale than those who claimed the opposite.
- Similar results can be observed for self-assessed health. The results for this variable, in Table 3.8a, suggest higher morale levels are associated with worsening health as perceived by the elderly respondents. Those who perceived their health to be good/excellent scored 0.17 points lower and those who perceived their health to be alright for their age scored 0.26 points lower, on the morale scale than those who perceived their health to be fair/poor, other characteristics being the same. This is contrary to expectations, in particular, where the more objective measures of physical health, 'physical health rating' and 'cumulative Pfeiffer score', suggest a health

effect on morale in the expected direction. This phenomenon may be due to complex relationships between the variables 'self-assessed health', 'friends in the area', omitted variables (e.g. frailty) and morale. This and other unexpected results are discussed further in subsequent sub-sections. A dubious assumption is relaxed in Sub-section 3.8.3. We suggest a method of controlling for the *time-variant* variables that were omitted from the analysis.

3.8.2.2. Past Behaviour or Markov Effect

Before proceeding to the discussion of the marginal likelihood method, we need to deal with the important issue of past behaviour. It is quite plausible that past high levels of morale may be indicative of present high levels of morale, i.e. that once high levels of morale are established, they tend to persist and vice versa; morale may be resistant to change. The only past observation on morale which is available in the NWEP is the observed level of morale at previous time points. Other measures such as duration in a state (e.g. low morale) are not available in the data set. In the analysis described in the previous section, no direct effects from past behaviour were assumed. We can include a past behaviour effect and test for it within the same modelling framework as the one described in previous section. A dummy variable representing past behaviour (i.e. morale level either in 1979 or in 1983) is included as an explanatory variable in each of the equations at times t and (t+1), respectively:

$$y_{it} = \beta_0 + \alpha y_{it-1} + \beta x_{it} + \theta_i + \varepsilon_{it} \tag{3.5}$$

$$y_{i(t+1)} = \beta_0 + \alpha y_{it} + \beta x_{i(t+1)} + \theta_i + \varepsilon_{i(t+1)} \tag{3.6}$$

Differencing equation (3.5) and (3.6) leads to :

$$y_{i(t+1)} - y_{it} = \alpha(y_{it} - y_{it-1}) + \beta(x_{i(t+1)} - x_{it}) + (\varepsilon_{i(t+1)} - \varepsilon_{it}) \tag{3.7}$$

This model can be fitted easily in the same way as described in the previous section. There are two important points that should be noted. First, as mentioned earlier, the survey observations in 1979 and 1983 enable us to test for past behaviour but this means that the analysis needs to be restricted to the 1983 and 1987 datasets. Second, fitting the model in equation (3.7) will lead to a well-known misspecification problem. This problem arises because equation (3.7) contains the terms y_{it} and ε_{it} on the right-hand side. This means that we have a model in which the error term ε_{it} is correlated with an included explanatory variable y_{it}. This leads to a serious specification problem. To demonstrate the effects of the specification problem, this model was fitted and the results suggested a significant negative association, i.e. previous low morale appeared to be indicative of present high morale and vice versa. This result is counterintuitive and highly implausible.

3.8.2.3. Error in Variables and Instrumental Variables

This problem is acknowledged specifically in the field of econometrics (e.g. see [19, 97, 99, 100]). The problem is often described in terms of measurement error and frequently referred to as 'error in variables' in the literature. This problem stems from variables that cannot be observed or measured precisely. For example, while age and sex may be precisely measured, state of health may not. The latter, in particular if self-assessed, will provide a combined measure of 'true' health and of error due to the respondents' state of well being at the time of the survey. In itself, this is not a major problem in an exploratory analysis involving crosstabulations. An awareness of the problem may assist with clarifying an exploratory study by introducing an intermediate category 'allright for age'. Such a distinction in measuring health indicates an appreciation of the problems associated with imprecise measurement. But it will not eradicate the problem of subjective measurements based on self-reporting.

However, the inclusion in the regression model of variables that are not precisely measured (or of variables measured with error) will cause model mis-specification and will breach the independence assumption. The problem arises because the error associated with some explanatory variables included in the model will be the source of an association between the included explanatory variables and the error term thereby violating the independence assumption. This problem can lead to erroneous results and misleading conclusions, and is referred to as the error-in-variables problem (see Appendix VIII).

This problem can be resolved with the application of *instrumental* variables. With this method, the offending variable(s) is replaced with another variable that is strongly correlated with the offending variable but which has no association with the regression error term.

3.8.2.4. Application of Instrumental Variables

We return to our specification problem with previous morale. Differencing had caused the presence of morale at 1983 (y_{it}) to appear in equation (3.7) through the term (y_{it}-y_{it-1}). To resolve this problem, we need to replace the dummy variable (y_{it}-y_{it-1}) with an instrumental variable that is not correlated with the error term but which is highly correlated with the dummy variable. The most straightforward choice of instrument variable that satisfies this criterion is morale in 1979. Therefore, we replaced (y_{it}-y_{it-1}) with y_{it-1} in equation (3.7). Interestingly, the model fitting results using instrumental variables offered no evidence that past behaviour is having a significant effect on morale (p=0.94).

There are computer packages that can handle such problems, for example, Time Series Processor (TSP), Shazam, HUMMER (see [19]), R, STATA, and SAS. For this exercise, TSP and HUMMER were used and produced similar results.

It can be seen from equations (4)-(6) in Appendix VIII that instrumental variables can be very useful in exploring complex relationships in survey data. This application is discussed further in Sub-section 3.8.3.

3.8.2.5. Marginal or Integrated Likelihood Method

In this section, we demonstrate the application of the model presented in Sub-section 3.7.1.3. As mentioned in Sub-section 3.7.2, morale is a continuous variable and thus the appropriate method to apply is the integrated likelihood method as described in Sub-section 3.7.1.3 (see Appendix VI). Any statistical package that offers the facility to fit random effects models, such as SAS, STATA, R and GENSTAT, may be used for the analysis presented here. We used VARCL[101]. The variable selection process is demonstrated in Tables 3.9 and 3.10, and the model fitting results are shown in Tables 3.11 and 3.12. Variables were tested in the model one at a time and their effect on morale was tested using the likelihood ratio test statistic (χ^2). Both Tables 3.9 and 3.10 show the deviance obtained at each step; the likelihood ratio test statistics are shown in brackets. The main feature of both tables is that the past behaviour effect appears not to be significant even on its own in stage 1 (column 3).

Table 3.9 suggests two possible models: one is to enter the dominant effect 'cumulative Pfeiffer score' in the model first; the second is to start with the 'physical health rating' variable. In the case of the first model, once the 'cumulative Pfeiffer score' has been entered in the model, all other objective variables become non-significant (Table 3.9, columns 4 and 5). Furthermore, 'cumulative Pfeiffer score' seems to control for the effects of the subjective measures (Table 3.9, column 5), i.e. those subjective variables which were significant on their own (column 3) are no longer significant. The log-likelihood for this model is -21.5. However, pursuing variable selection with 'physical health rating' in the model first results in a slightly different model; for the objective model, the variable 'mental health rating' is now significant at the 10% level (Table 3.10, column 3). The objective model therefore includes both physical and mental health ratings. The inclusion of subjective measures in the modelling process begins with the 'physical health rating' being added to the model first. This variable seems to control for all the remaining variables, including the subjective measures which were significant on their own, with the exception of 'confidant'. The inclusion of this subjective variable in the model means that the 'mental health rating' variable is no longer significant. The log-likelihood for this model is -24.29 indicating a slightly poorer fit despite the presence of 'cumulative Pfeiffer score' and 'Pfeiffer Scale: Physical health rating' in the model. The two models have been fitted separately and their results are shown in Tables 3.11 and 3.12.

Table 3.9. Variable selection process for the marginal likelihood method - α at the 5% level* (N=38)

Stages of the analysis		Stage 1 - Model of objective variables		2 - Add subjective variables
Explanatory variables	d.f	Deviance (L.R)	Deviance (L.R)	Deviance (L.R)
Null/restricted model		68.75	43.00	
Markov effect	1	67.90 (.85)		
Objective measures				
Frequency see family	4	66.84 (1.91)	-	
Relative seen most	3	65.46 (3.30)	-	
Household composition	2	65.00 (3.75)	-	
Has close relatives	1	66.89 (1.87)	-	
Isolation measure	1	66.67 (2.10)	-	
Home tenure	2	66.86 (1.89)	-	
Network type	4	62.27 (6.48)	-	
Income	3	65.50 (3.30)	-	
Housebound	1	65.00 (3.75)	42.34 (0.66)	
Number of years widow	1	68.23 (0.51)	-	
Visit relatives	3	63.60 (5.17)	-	
Age	1	68.64 (0.11)	-	
Have a phone	1	68.00 (0.75)	-	
Hours spent alone	2	64.78 (3.97)	-	
Nearest neighbour	1	67.38 (1.37)	-	
Pfeiffer Scale:				
Social rating scale	1	61.14 (7.61)	42.20 (0.80)	
Mental health rating	1	58.85 (9.90)	42.30 (0.70)	
Physical health rating	1	54.97 (13.78)	42.93 (0.07)	
Activities of daily living	1	62.37 (6.38)	40.97 (2.03)	
Economic resources	1	66.90 (1.85)		
Cumulative Pfeiffer score	1	43.00 (25.75)	INCLUDED	INCLUDED
Marital status (m.s.)	2	67.11 (1.64)	-	
Change in m.s.	1	66.65 (2.10)	-	
Subjective measures				
Presence of friends	1	68.60 (0.15)		-
People do favours	2	66.90 (1.85)		-

Stages of the analysis	Stage 1 - Model of objective variables		2 - Add subjective variables
Self-assessed health	2	59.30 (9.45)	42.75 (0.25)
Health limited activities	1	63.70 (5.05)	42.89 (0.11)
Confidant	2	59.14 (9.61)	41.70 (1.30)
Wish for more friends	1	67.00 (1.77)	
Log-likelihood		-21.5	-21.5

* Values in brackets are the deviance for the added variable e.g. for the first round (deviance of null model – deviance of the variable). A typical VARCL output prints deviance (D) for fitted model.

Table 3.10. Alternative variable selection process for the marginal likelihood method - α at the 5% level* - (N=38)

Stages of the analysis		Stage 1 - Model of objective variables			Stage 2 - Add subjective variables	
Explanatory variables	d.f	Deviance (L.R)	Deviance (L.R)	Deviance (L.R)	Deviance (L.R)	Deviance (L.R)
Null/restricted model		68.75	54.97	52.13	54.97	48.57
Markov effect		67.90 (0.85)				
Objective measures						
Frequency see family	4	66.84 (1.91)	-			
Relative seen most	3	65.46 (3.30)	-			
Household composition	2	65.00 (1.32)	-			
Has close relatives	1	66.89 (1.87)	-			
Isolation measure	1	66.67 (2.10)	-			
Home tenure	2	66.86 (1.89)	-			
Network type	4	62.27 (6.48)	-			
Income	3	65.50 (3.30)	-			
Housebound	1	65.00 (3.75)	53.40 (1.57)	-		
Number of years widow	1	68.23 (0.51)	-			
Visit relatives	3	63.60 (5.17)	-			
Age	1	68.64 (0.11)	-			
Have a phone	1	68.00 (0.75)	-			
Hours spent alone	2	64.78 (3.97)	-			
Nearest neighbour	1	67.38 (1.37)	-			
Pfeiffer Scale:						
Social rating scale	1	61.14 (7.61)	53.02 (1.95)	-		
Mental health rating	1	58.85 (9.90)	52.13 (2.84)	INCLUDED	52.13 (2.84)	-
Physical health rating	1	54.97 (13.78)	INCLUDED	INCLUDED	INCLUDED	INCLUDED
Activities of daily living	1	62.37 (6.38)	54.83 (0.14)	-		
Economic resources	1	66.90 (1.85)	-			
Cumulative Pfeiffer score	1	43.00 (25.75)	EXCLUDED	EXCLUDED	EXCLUDED	EXCLUDED
Marital status (m.s.)	2	67.11 (1.64)	-			
Change in m.s.	2	66.65 (2.10)	-			
Subjective measures						
Presence of friends	1	68.60 (0.15)			-	
People do favours	2	66.90 (1.85)			-	
Self-assessed health	2	59.30 (9.45)			51.34 (0.79)	-
Health limited activities	1	63.70 (5.05)			52.10 (0.03)	-
Confidant	2	59.14 (9.61)			48.57 (6.40)	INCLUDED
Wish for more friends	1	67.00 (1.77)			-	
Log-likelihood				-26.6		-24.29

* Values in brackets are the deviance for the added variable e.g. for the first round (deviance of null model – deviance of the variable). A typical VARCL output prints deviance (D) for fitted model.

The results for the marginal likelihood analysis seem to confirm the role of physical health throughout the analysis whether measured as self-assessed health, more objectively as 'physical health rating' or as a cumulative dependency measure. The high within-individual correlations (R^2 of 0.66 and 0.42 from Tables 3.11 and 3.12 respectively) emphasize the importance of adopting a methodology which allows control for residual heterogeneity.

Clearly, physical health and dependency appear to influence morale. Those with higher physical health dependency (as measured by the Pfeiffer physical health score), on average, score 0.15 points lower on the morale scale (other characteristics being the same). The results for the variable 'confidant' are not unexpected: those with a confidant appear to score higher on the morale scale than those who claimed they had no confidant. Those elderly individuals with a spouse as their confidant appear to do better.

Table 3.11. Marginal likelihood method - Model fitting results (1983-87) - Model 1

Explanatory variables	Estimates	Standard Errors
Grand Mean	3.08	0.05
Objective variables		
Cumulative Pfeiffer Score	-0.05	0.01
Log-likelihood	-21.5	

Estimate of Variance components			
	Variance	Sigma	Standard Error for Sigma
Intervals (ε_{it})	0.04	0.21	
Individual (θ_i)	0.08	0.28	0.04
Deviance	43.00		

$$R^2 = \frac{(\sigma_\theta)^2}{(\sigma_\theta)^2+(\sigma_\varepsilon)^2} = \frac{0.08}{0.08+0.04} = 0.66$$

Table 3.12. Marginal likelihood method - Model fitting results (1983-87) - Model 2

Explanatory variables	Estimates	Standard Errors
Grand Mean	2.66	0.05
Objective variables		
Physical health rating	-0.15	0.04
Subjective variables		
Confidant		
No-one	0.00	
Spouse	0.38	0.15
Other	0.20	0.12
Log-likelihood	-24.29	

Estimate of Variance components			
	Variance	Sigma	Standard error for Sigma
Intervals (ε_{it})	0.07	0.26	
Individual (θ_i)	0.05	0.23	0.05
Deviance	48.57		

$$R^2 = \frac{(\sigma_\theta)^2}{(\sigma_\theta)^2+(\sigma_\varepsilon)^2} = \frac{0.05}{0.05+0.07} = 0.42$$

3.8.3. Controlling for Time-Variant Omitted Variables: Instrumental Variables Revisited

The longitudinal modelling discussed so far has concentrated on controlling for time-constant omitted heterogeneity (θ_i). In studies of social processes, the effects from time-variant omitted variables may also be present, e.g. the 'feel good' factor. We could conceptualise a 'variance component' model to account explicitly for the time-variant omitted variables as follows:

$$y_{it} = \beta_0 + \beta x_{it} + \zeta_{it}$$

or

$$y_{it} = \beta_0 + \beta x_{it} + \theta_i + \xi_{it} + \varepsilon_{it} \tag{3.8}$$

where $\zeta = \theta + \xi + \varepsilon$; θ is the time-constant omitted heterogeneity, ξ is the time-variant omitted variable, and ε is the i.i.d. random error term. We could write another equation for the next time point, i.e. (t+1), but before we go any further, note that, with this conceptualisation, in addition to the usual parameters and structural error term, we have two additional nuisance parameters. Remember that dealing with only one additional nuisance parameter which is time-constant (θ) was not an easy task. Controlling for two additional nuisance parameters, one of which is time-variant, will be an even bigger problem to overcome. However, in this book we show a novel method of controlling for both time-constant and time-variant parameters simultaneously.

The approach will be similar to the conditional and marginal methods discussed in the previous section, namely, eliminating the nuisance parameter from the equation. In the proposed method, we eliminate both parameters using instrumental variables. The conceptualisation of this application is shown in Appendix IX, also see [63].

The approach works on the premise that the analysis includes explanatory variable(s) that have not been measured precisely and that these variable(s) have been identified. Reconsider the analysis of morale in old age. The data for this analysis were generated from a social survey and the explanatory variables were classed according to their measurement bias as 'true' measures and 'imprecise' measures which we termed objective and subjective variables respectively. Recall that, because of the nature of the measurements, the subjective variables were the sources of model mis-specification. Therefore, to tackle this problem, we could incorporate instrumental variables into the modelling framework reported in Sub-section 3.8.2.1. In other words, we could use the *objective* variables, which are significant and selected for inclusion in the model, as *instruments* for the subjective variables in the model– see Appendix IX.

In order to achieve simultaneous control for time-constant and time-variant nuisance parameters, the approach described in Appendix IX is based on the following principles:-

1. Identifiable imprecise measurements (variables)
2. Applicability of methods of conditioning or integrating out nuisance parameters (i.e. availability of longitudinal data)

3. Availability and applicability of instrumental variables

Each variable has already been identified as subjective or objective, and there are data available on at least two time points. From the earlier discussion of past behaviour (Subsections 3.4.3 and 3.8.2.2) on we know that the application of instrumental variables is necessary and that variables are available in the NWEP dataset to be used as *instruments*. Therefore, to use the approach described in Appendix IX, the conditional likelihood method for a continuous response variable was repeated. However, after conditioning data on the sufficient statistic ($y_{it}-y_{it-1}$), we subjected the model to the application of instrumental variables. In other words, the statistically significant objective variables selected for inclusion in the model were used as *instruments* for the statistically significant subjective variables included in the model. In doing so, we are effectively estimating the model conceptualised in equation (3.8).

Note also that using the objective variables as instruments to estimate the subjective variables is equivalent to conducting stages 2 and 3 of the pragmatic approach (Figure 3.1). A parsimonious model based on the objective variables was selected, and the variables from this model were then used as instruments for the subjective variables. As mentioned in Subsection 3.8.2.4, the technique of instrumental variables can be conducted using available software such as Time Series Processor (TSP), Shazam, HUMMER (see [19]), R, STATA, LIMDEP, NLOGIT and SAS. Variable selection and model fitting were carried out in HUMMER [19] and the results are shown in Tables 3.13 and 3.14 respectively.

Table 3.13. Variable selection process using conditional likelihood method and instrumental variables - p-values given below are for F-ratio goodness of test statistic; α= 10% level (N=38)

Explanatory variables	Stage 1- Objective variables only			Stage 2 - instrument	
		Model 1	Model 2	Model 1	Model 2
Markov effect	0.94				
Objective measures					
Frequency see family	0.23	-	-	-	-
Relative seen most	0.32	-	-	-	-
Household composition	0.32	-	-	-	-
Has close relatives	0.05	0.03	IN	-	IN*
Isolation measure	0.44	-	-	-	-
Home tenure	0.88	-	-	-	-
Network type	0.17	-	-	-	-
Income	0.44	-	-	-	-
Bedfast	0.18	-	-	-	-
Number of years widow	0.37	-	-	-	-
Visit relatives	0.87	-	-	-	-
Age	0.89	-	-	-	-
Have a phone	0.32	-	-	-	-
Hours spent alone	0.01	IN	0.01	0.01	IN*	IN*
Nearest neighbour	0.25	-	-	-	-
Pfeiffer Scale:					
Social rating scale	0.06	0.07	-	0.66	-
Mental health rating	0.22	-	-	-	-
Physical health rating	0.17	-	-	-	-
Activities of daily living	0.17	-	-	-	-
Economic resources	0.20	-	-	-	-
Cumulative Pfeiffer score	0.045	0.06	0.15	IN	-	IN*
Marital status (m.s)	0.51	-	-	-	-
Change in change in m.s.	0.78	-	-	-	-

Explanatory variables	Stage 1- Objective variables only			Stage 2 - instrument	
		Model 1	Model 2	Model 1	Model 2
Subjective measures					
Presence of friends	0.01			IN	IN
People do favours	0.65			-	-
Self-assessed health	0.015			-	-
Health limited activities	0.87			-	-
Confidant	0.13			-	-
Wish for more friends	0.3			-	-
R-squared		0.30	0.29	0.34	0.22

* These variables were used as instruments.

Variable selection proceeds as previously with a bivariate analysis (Table 3.13, stage 1). This stage does not involve instrumental variables and therefore the results should be very similar to the first stage of variable selection using the conditional likelihood method. The results are reassuringly very close, to two decimal places, to those of Table 3.7. By stage 2, it becomes obvious that there may be two possible alternative models: one with 'hours spent alone' and 'has close relative', and the other model with 'hours spent alone' and 'cumulative Pfeiffer score'. Now we have two possible models of morale in old age based entirely on the objective variables. The subjective variables are in part controlled for or, in effect, are influenced by the objective variables. The instrumental variable method fits a regression of the subjective variables 'presence of friends in the area' and 'self-assessed state of health' on the objective variables included in the model of stage one. The predicted values from this regression are used in a regression of morale on both the selected objective and subjective variables. As a result, the variable 'self-assessed health' was no longer significant. This suggests that 'self-assessed health' has very little effect on morale. Therefore, the variable 'self-assessed health' was dropped from the model. This lends support to an earlier discussion (Sub-section 3.8.2.1) on subjective variables such as 'self-assessed health' that these variables are associated with omitted variables other than 'frailty' which was already accounted for. The model fitting results are shown in Table 3.14.

After controlling for the time-variant omitted variables, the subjective variable 'presence of friends in the area' is also affected. This variable, which was highly significant in both Tables 3.8a and 3.8b, is now only significant at the 20% level in model 1 and is no longer significant in model 2 (Table 3.14). Unlike the results from the conditional likelihood method on its own, now model 2, which includes the variable 'has close relatives', appears to be a better fit than model 1.

The results of model 2 in Table 3.14 imply that those spending less than 3 hours on their own do better than others on the morale scale, including those spending more than 9 hours on their own. Although this variable was suggested to be a proxy for dependence due to physical illness in the previous analysis, now *some* of the quality of life associated with it is reflected by this result. It is plausible that those who spend less than 3 hours on their own are the married respondents, and that those who spend more than 9 hours on their own are less dependent, more mobile and require less looking after. Those who tend to spend 3-9 hours on their own are likely to be those more dependent respondents who require more looking after. This group appears to do worse on the morale scale. There are three points to note from Table 3.14. The first is that the estimated effect for the variable 'has close relatives' is reassuringly in the expected direction; those who claimed to have no living close relatives score 0.32 points lower on the morale scale than those who said they did have living close relatives. The second point is that, as discussed above, the variable 'friends in the area' is no longer significant, suggesting that it owed its significant association with morale to its association with an unobserved variable. The third point is that the results in this table seem to suggest that, over time, morale in old age may be seen more as a function of levels of dependency, and that a lack of close relatives (possibly to rely on or to relate to) exacerbates the situation.

Table 3.14. Model fitting results using conditional likelihood method and instrumental variables - (N=38)

Explanatory variables	Models			
Objective measures	Model 1		Model 2	
	p.e.	s.e.	p.e.	s.e.
Hours spent alone				
Up to 3 hours	-0.11	0.27	0.11	0.18
3-9 hours	-0.39	0.20	-0.37	0.14
More than 9 hours	0.00		0.00	
Pfeiffer scale				
Cumulative score	-0.04	0.02		
Has close relatives				
Yes			0.00	
No			-0.32	0.13
Subjective measures				
Presence of friends				
Yes	0.00		0.00	
No	1.44	1.06	0.22	0.64
R-squared	0.22		0.34	

3.8.4. Concluding Remarks

One of the issues to be addressed in this book (see Chapter 1) is to assess the insight gained from applying progressively complex models to data. In doing so, we raised awareness of the relationship between complexity in methodology and the substantive issues. For example, do we gain more insight if we apply complex data drenching methods to analyse cross-sectional data than the pragmatic approach demonstrated in the cross-sectional analysis sections (3.6 and 3.7)? Indeed we may gain more understanding of the topic under investigation with the application of the latter. This is because the pragmatic approach explicitly addresses the important substantive issues during the analysis and interpretation of results. A relevant issue is therefore appropriateness of methodology, e.g. not only is no insight gained but also we may produce erroneous results if we apply complex cross-sectional methods to longitudinal data. And clearly, we may arrive at misleading conclusions as a result of the mis-application of statistical methodology. To complete the demonstration of various methodologies, we will compare the various statistical models, the results of which are reproduced in Table 3.15. The complexities arose from a desire to control for additional sources of variation and to take into account additional information. The main reason for wanting to increase model complexity was to investigate change over time in the social process under investigation, namely morale in old age. Consequently, longitudinal data or repeated observations on the process are required, thereby increasing the ability to control for past behaviour effects and residual heterogeneity. Intuitively, it is expected that the ability to control for additional sources of variation, and to account for more information, will lead to additional insight into the process. However, the association between longitudinal data and the additional flexibility to incorporate control into the analysis should not be confused with ignoring the main issues associated with the dynamics of human behaviour when dealing with cross-sectional data. These issues can be incorporated implicitly and pragmatically when conducting analyses and interpreting results, as in the cross-sectional analyses presented in Sections 3.6 and 3.7.

In order to disentangle the complex inter-relationships between variables within the statistical modelling framework, it is necessary to control for various sources of variation. As shown in Figure 3.3, with the cross-sectional methodology the best that could be done to achieve this was: (i) to distinguish between objective and subjective variables, and (ii) to pool the 1983 and 1987 data. The pragmatic approach discussed in Section 3.6 was to use the subjective/objective classification to investigate intra-individual variation in the data *implicitly*, i.e. to interpret the subjective variables as either intervening or independent effects. The results from the pooled cross-sectional analysis suggested that the subjective variable 'confidant' may have an intervening rather than a direct effect on morale, over and above the objective variable 'Pfeiffer: physical health'. The analysis is summarised in the second column of Table 3.15. The longitudinal methodology permits *explicit* control for the intra-individual variation or residual heterogeneity. The results from the longitudinal models are presented in columns 3, 4, 5 and 6 of Table 3.15. The application of different methods applied to the morale data is summarized in Figure 3.3.

The model fitting results from the pooled cross-sectional method can be directly compared with the results from the marginal likelihood method (see model 2, column 6, Table 3.15). It can be seen that, after controlling for the residual heterogeneity, the effect of the subjective variable 'confidant' is substantially reduced. The parameter estimate reflects this effect. Note also that the effect of the variable 'Pfeiffer physical health' is marginally reduced.

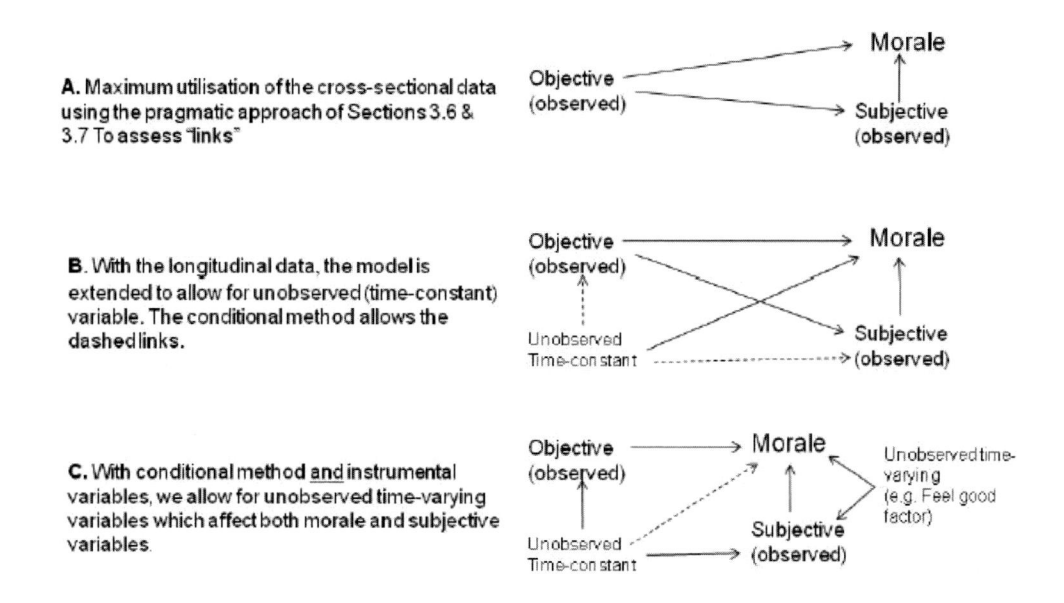

Figure 3.3. Graphical representation of level of control imposed by each methodology.

Table 3.15. Summary of results from pooled cross-sectional and longitudinal analyses of morale data

	Cross-sectional pooled		Longitudinal													
			Conditional				Marginal				Conditional and Instrumental variables					
			Model 1		Model 2		Model 1		Model 2		Model 1		Model 2	
	p.e.	s.e.	p.e.	s.e.	p.e.	s.e.	p.e.	s.e.	p.e.	s.e.	p.e.	s.e.	p.e.	s.e.
Objective variables														
Pfeiffer - physical rating	-0.18	0.04							-0.15	0.04				
Pfeiffer - mental rating														
Pfeiffer - cumulative			-0.03	0.01			-0.05	0.01			-0.04	0.02		
Hours spend alone														
More than 9 hours			0.00		(0.00)						0.00		0.00	
3-9 hours			-0.34	0.12	(-0.38)	(0.13)					-0.39	0.20	-0.37	0.14
Up to 3 hours			0.04	0.13	(0.07)	(0.13)					-0.11	0.27	0.11	0.18
Has close relatives														
Yes					(0.00)								0.00	
No					(-0.32)	(0.13)							-0.32	0.13
Subjective variables														
Self-assessed health														
Fair/poor			0.00											
Alright			-0.26	0.11										
Excellent/good			-0.17	0.15										
Confidant														
No one	0.00								0.00					
Spouse	0.54	0.15							0.38	0.15				
Other	0.32	0.13							0.20	0.12				
Presence of friends														
Yes			0.00		(0.00)						0.00		0.00	
No			0.46	0.15	(0.43)	(0.15)					1.44	1.06	0.22	0.64

The values in parentheses are the results of fitting the model excluding 'cumulative Pfeiffer score' and 'self-assessed health' which appears to be a poorer fit (R^2=0.44 compared to R^2=0.56 for model 1, Tables 3.8a and 3.8b).

On the other hand, the conditional likelihood method, which does not assume independence, produced different results. With the conditional likelihood method, the inter-relationships between omitted and explanatory variables are taken into account by conditioning omitted variables out of the model. The conditional likelihood method identifies more significant explanatory variables than the cross-sectional and the marginal likelihood methods. The health and dependency effects are handled more explicitly with model 1 of the conditional method (Table 3.8a), i.e. through the presence of the variables 'Pfeiffer cumulative score', 'self-assessed health' and, at least in part, 'hours alone'. The mental competence effect can be interpreted through the presence of variables 'presence of friend' and 'Pfeiffer cumulative score'. The alternative model, model 2, which is a poorer fit, appears to suggest that companionship from close relatives, including spouse, may be related to high morale in old age. As discussed earlier (e.g. see Sub-section 3.8.2.2), any companionship effects measured by variables such as 'hours alone', 'presence of friend' and 'close living relative' may be compounded with perceptions of help at hand. Therefore, in effect, both models suggest that poorer health and dependency are inversely related to morale in old age.

The model fitting results using the conditional likelihood method appear to suggest that the subjective variables are predominantly related to morale as independent effects. There are only small changes in the parameter estimates of the objective model after including the subjective variables. However, anomalous results could also be seen in the parameter estimates of 'self-assessed health' and in particular 'presence of friend': the counter intuitive results, that low morale is associated with good health and availability of friends, are unexpected! This suggests that controlling for time-constant residual heterogeneity may not be sufficient, and there may be other relationships in the data which have not been accounted for. The use of the conditional likelihood method, together with instrumental variables, introduced in the latter part of this chapter, allows control for time-variant omitted variables simultaneously with other structural and nuisance parameters. There are computational difficulties with the application of instrumental variables within the marginal likelihood modelling framework which need to be identified and resolved. One of the main drawbacks with the marginal method is that it assumes the error term to be independent of the explanatory variables.

The results shown in the final two columns of Table 3.15 suggest that the subjective variables are no longer significant. Moreover, the results can be interpreted as low morale being associated with physical dependence on 'others', while the availability of, or (both physical and mental) dependence on, close relatives including spouse may lead to high morale in old age.

Finally, because of more extensive control, the final analyses have more authority but all the results reported do tend to emphasize the complexity of the task in developing parsimonious models when there is high multicollinearity between variables. An additional advantage with the final analyses over the conditional likelihood method is to allow the inclusion of time-invariant factors in the modelling process. For example, the effects from time-constant variables such as sex could be controlled for after differencing by using such variables as instruments for subjective variables which are known to carry measurement error.

Chapter 4

SABRE

4.1. INTRODUCTION

As the name SABRE (Software for the Analysis of Binary Recurrent Events) suggests, this software was developed to fill a void in statistical computing left by commercial and specialist software to handle multi-process events and response sequences. SABRE enables the researcher to control for residual heterogeneity (or omitted variables) when modelling survey data. Clearly, the availability of computer software that allows control for additional sources of variation not previously accounted for should, at least in theory, encourage wider utilisation of models that were mathematically more complex.

Since its initial version in 1989, SABRE has grown considerably. Its current version (6.0) enables the analysis of multi-process event/response sequences i.e. it is capable of fitting a number of different models to data depending on the nature of the outcome variable(s). In other words, SABRE can handle the simple binary outcomes (yes/no), multinomial or ordinal outcomes (e.g. describing state of health as excellent, good, allright, poor), and bivariate binary where the response may comprise a pair of binary outcomes – see examples in the next chapter. For more details see http://www.lancs.ac.uk/staff/cpajp/SABRE/index.html.

In summary, SABRE can fit models with the following specifications:-

- Fits the mover-stayer model, conventional logistic, logistic-normal and logistic-normal with end-points models to binary data, e.g. studies of voting behaviour, trade union membership, economic activity and migration.
- Fits the ordered probit and logit random effect response models e.g. studies of voting behaviour, trade union membership, economic activity and migration.
- Fits conventional log-linear, log-linear normal and log-linear normal with end-point models to count data, e.g. demographic surveys.
- Substantial control is available over the parameters of the algorithm for the sophisticated user, e.g. studies of infertility in humans.
- Can deal with very long sequences of data, e.g. animal husbandry.
- Can deal with multi-process data, where each response sequence is of a different type, currently limited to the simultaneous analysis of trivariate correlated sequences, e.g. animal husbandry, e.g. absenteeism studies, clustered sampling schemes.

- Comprehensive online user manual. and online training materials.

Section 4.2 provides a description of the modelling capability of SABRE. For a full discussion of the mathematical models which can be fitted in SABRE, the interested reader is also referred to Crouchley and Berridge [102]. Readers may choose to skip the next section and go straight to installing SABRE (Section 4.3) and to the examples illustrating how to run SABRE (Sections 4.4 and 4.5) including sample runs for the applications described in Chapter 5.

4.2. STATISTICAL MODELS IN SABRE

SABRE is a program for the statistical analysis of multi-process event/response sequences. These responses can take the form of binary, ordinal, count and continuoous recurrent events. The response sequences can also be combinations of different types (e.g. continuous [wages] and binary [trade union membership]). Such multi-process data are common in many research areas, e.g. in the analysis of work and life histories from the British Household Panel Survey or the German Socio-Economic Panel Study where researchers often want to disentangle state dependence (the effect of previous responses or related outcomes) from any omitted effects that might be present in recurrent behaviour (e.g. unemployment).

SABRE can also be used to model collections of single sequences such as may occur in medical trials, e.g. headaches and epileptic seizures [103, 104], or clustered cross-sectional data such as the educational attainment of children in schools. The class of models that can be estimated by SABRE may be called Multivariate Generalised Linear Mixed Models. These models have special features added to the standard multilevel models to help them disentangle state dependence from the incidental parameters (omitted or unobserved effects). The incidental parameters can be treated as random or fixed, the random effects models being estimated using standard Gaussian quadrature or adaptive **Gaussian quadrature. 'End effects' can also be added to the models to accommodate 'stayers' or 'non-susceptibles'.** The fixed effects algorithm that has been developed for SABRE uses code for large sparse matrices from the Harwell Subroutine Library, see *http://www.cse.scitech.ac.uk/nag/hsl/*.

SABRE also includes the option to undertake all of the calculations using increased accuracy. This is important because numerical underflow and overflow often occur in the estimation process for models with incidental parameters. This feature does not seem to be available in other similar software: -

1. http://cran.r-project.org/web/packages/lme4/index.html
2. http://cran.r-project.org/web/packages/npmlreg/index.html
3. http://www.stata.com/
4. http://www.gllamm.org/
5. http://www.sas.com/

4.2.1. Event History Models

An important type of discrete data occurs when modelling the duration to some pre-specified event such as the duration in unemployment from the start of a spell of unemployment until the start of work, the time between shopping trips, or the time to first marriage. This type of discrete data has several important features. For instance, the durations or times to the events of interest are often not observed for all the sampled subjects or individuals. This often happens because the event of interest had not happened by the end of the observation window; when this happens we say that the spell was right censored.

The second important feature of social science duration data is that the temporal scale of most social processes is so large (months/years) that it is inappropriate to assume that the explanatory variables remain constant, e.g. in an unemployment spell, the local labour market unemployment rate will vary (at the monthly level) as the local and national economic conditions change. Other explanatory variables, like the subjects' age, change automatically with time.

The third important feature of social science duration data occurs when the observation window cuts into an ongoing spell; this is called left censoring. We will assume throughout that left censoring is non-informative for event history models. The first three features of social science duration data can be accommodated using two- and three-level binary response models in SABRE.

The fourth important feature of duration data is that the spells can be of different types, e.g. the duration of a household in rented accommodation, until they move to another rented property, could have different characteristics to the duration of a household in rented accommodation until they become owner occupiers. This type of data can be modelled using competing risk models using multivariate generalised linear (binary response) models in SABRE (see www.SABRE.lancs.ac.uk).

In social science duration data, we typically observe a spell over a sequence of intervals, e.g. weeks or months, so SABRE concentrates on methods for discrete-time data. We are not reducing our modelling options by doing this, as durations measured at finer intervals of time such as days, hours, or even seconds can also be written out as a sequence of intervals. We can also group the data by using larger intervals (such as weeks or months) than those over which the durations are measured.

Event history data occur when we observe repeated duration events. If these events are of the same type, we have renewal data which can be modelled using univariate generalised linear (binary response) models in SABRE.

4.2.2. Stayers, Nonsusceptibles and Endpoints

There are empirical situations in which a subset of the population behaves differently to those that follow the proposed generalised linear model. For instance, in a migration study, we could observe a large group of individuals who do not move or migrate from a region over the study period. These observed non-migrators could be made up of two distinct groups: (i) those that consider migrating, but are not observed to do so during the observation period; (ii) those that would never consider migrating (stayers). This phenomenon can occur in various modelling contexts, e.g. in the zero-inflated Poisson model [105], in the mover-stayer model

[106] and in the competing risk context, where the data could come from a population that consists of some subjects who are susceptible and others who are nonsusceptible to the event of interest.

It has also often been noted that the goodness-of-fit of mixture models like generalised linear mixed models can be improved by adding a spike to the parametric distribution for the random effects to explicitly represent stayers, giving 'spiked distributions' [107]. Non-parametric representations of the random effects distribution [108], (see e.g. Davies and Crouchley [109]), have the flexibility to accommodate stayers. However, non-parametric random effects distributions can require a lot of parameters (mass point locations and probabilities) to be estimated. Spiked distributions are available for binary response and Poisson models in SABRE.

4.2.3. State Dependence

State dependence was discussed in Chapter 1 and subsequently in Chapter 3 when dealing with longitudinal data. Longitudinal and panel data on recurrent events are substantively important in social science research for two reasons. First, they provide some scope for extending control for variables that have been omitted from the analysis. For example, differencing, as demonstrated in Subsections 3.8.1 and 3.8.2.1, provides a simple way of removing time constant effects (both omitted and observed) from the analysis. Second, a distinctive feature of social science theory is that it postulates that behaviour and outcomes are typically influenced by previous behaviour and outcomes (e.g. see Figure 3.3), that is, there is positive `feedback' (e.g. the McGinnis [110]) `axiom of cumulative inertia'). A frequently noted empirical regularity in the analysis of unemployment data is that those who were unemployed in the past or who have worked in the past are more likely to be unemployed (or working) in the future (Heckman [111], p. 706). Is this due to a causal effect of being unemployed (or working) or is it a manifestation of a stable trait (random effect)?

Most observational schemes for collecting panel and other longitudinal data commence with the process already under way. They will therefore tend to have an informative start; the initial observed response is typically dependent upon pre-sample outcomes and unobserved variables. In contrast to time series analysis and, as explained by Anderson and Hsiao [97], Heckman [11, 112], Bhargava and Sargan [113] and others, failure to allow for this informative start, when state dependence and random effects are present, will prejudice consistent parameter estimation. Various treatments of the initial conditions problem for recurrent events with state dependence and random effects have been proposed, e.g. see [104, 114-117]. SABRE allows for these treatments in generalised linear models which incorporate first order state dependence.

4.2.4. Linear Model with Fixed Effects

The main objective of the random effects/multilevel modelling approach considered so far has been the estimation of regression parameters in the presence of random effects or incidental parameters. This has been done by assuming that the incidental parameters are Gaussian distributed and by computing the expected behaviour of individuals randomly sampled from this distribution (in other words, by integrating the random effects out of the model). This approach will provide consistent estimates of the regression parameters so long as, in the true model, the random effects are independent of the covariates.

An alternative approach is to estimate the model parameters by the usual maximum likelihood procedures using dummy variables for the incidental parameters. Hsiao ([118], Section 3.2) shows that, by using dummy variables for the incidental parameters, in a linear model with time-varying covariates, we get the same estimates as those of the time demeaned model. SABRE has a fixed effects estimator for the linear model.

4.3. INSTALLING AND USING SABRE

SABRE 6 is a stand-alone package and can be downloaded as a compressed file from http://www.lancs.ac.uk/staff/cpajp/SABRE/SABREform.php. It is free but users are required to fill in a registration form and are given the option of becoming a member of the SABRE user community. Once unpacked, SABRE is ready to use. It is an interactive program but it is easy to run batch files and to store the results in an output file.

To run SABRE, double click on the SABRE icon. SABRE then opens a DOS window in which SABRE may be used interactively or, alternatively, batch files may be run.

For a list of SABRE commands, see Appendix X.

4.4. EXAMPLE OF A SAMPLE RUN

Important components of a statistical analysis are a data set and the variables it contains. In a typical analysis in SABRE, data need to be identified before you can perform an analysis. In SABRE, a list of variables needs to be issued first so that SABRE associates each column in the data set with a variable name. Then, data must be read in using the 'read' command.

In an interactive session, data may be typed in or read from a data file. It may be more convenient to prepare the analysis in an ASCII text file and run commands in SABRE as a batch file. As an example, the following set of commands was input into SABRE as a batch file:

```
c
c create output file
c

out result.txt

c ccccccccccccccccccccccccccccccccccccccccc
c                                         c
c model fitting for Disability in the family c
c                                         c
c yvar is ybhard==1 hardship                 c
c                                         c
c ==0 low/no family hardship                 c
```

```
c                                              c
c                                              c
c ccccccccccccccccccccccccccccccccccccccccc

data serialno sex age  sh ill smok &
 disabl ybhard

read w3w7.dat

caseid serialno
fac sex fsex
fac sh fsh
fac smok fsmo
fac ill fill
fac disabl fdisab

hist ybhard

endpoints both

constant cons

yvar ybhard

c ccccccccc
c
c fit the null model
c
c ccccccccccccccccccccccccccc

fit cons
dis m

c cccccccccccccc
c
c model 1 add disability to the null model
c
c cccccccccccccccccccc


fit cons fdisabl
dis m
dis e
```
***

All the lines beginning with c are comments and are not executed by SABRE. So the first comment provides information about the first command line which instructs SABRE to create an output file and route the results from the screen into this file.

The next comment provides more information about what is being modeled, i.e the response variable and its values.

The data command tells SABRE the list and order of variables to be read from the data file. The & is a command line continuation indicator.

The read command reads the data from the data file called w3w7.dat. The data file must have a case identifier such as a case number variable. The next command tells SABRE that the case identifier is the first variable called serialno.

The factor command (fac) is used to declare the categorical variables.

The command hist on the next line generates a histogram of the response variable which is useful not only to get an idea of the distribution but also to detect any anomalies in the data.

The endpoints command tells SABRE to fit a mover-stayer model and to include both endpoints.

The constant command declares 'cons' to be the variable to be used as the regression intercept and yvar declares the variable ybhar to be the response variable.

Fit cons fits a null model with no explanatory variables included. This is particularly useful as a baseline against which to assess the goodness of fit of models which include explanatory variables. The display (dis) command will display details of fitting a model: dis m will provide model fitting details including convergence criteria and deviance, and dis e will display parameter estimates and standard errors.

4.5. SABRE APPLICATIONS FOR THIS BOOK

The simplest statistical model can be generalized to handle more complex scenarios. In the current context, we have already seen how the standard binary logistic regression model for cross-sectional binary outcomes can be generalized in various ways in order to analyse longitudinal binary data:

i. individual-specific random error can be added to the model in order to handle residual heterogeneity (see Sub-section 5.2.1.4);
ii. the mover-stayer model can be incorporated into the modelling framework (see Sub-section 5.2.1.4).

In Sub-section 4.5.1, we demonstrate how SABRE may be used to fit the binary logistic random effects model by way of an application to the teenage smoking data introduced here and described in more detail in Section 5.2. The binary logistic random effects model itself may be generalized in any number of ways. In this book, we concentrate attention on two possible generalizations:

a   First, we generalize from a single repeated outcome comprising two categories to a single repeated response which consists of more than two categories that are inherently ordered in some sense. A classical example of such a response is the Likert item [119] which comprises the categories: 'strongly agree', 'agree', 'neither agree nor disagree', 'disagree', 'strongly disagree'. The ordinal logistic (or cumulative logit) model [54] with random effects may be used to analyse repeated ordered categorical data.

b   Second, we generalize from a single repeated outcome to two repeated responses. An additional requirement of an appropriate model is the ability to assess the degree to which the two responses are correlated with each other. A classic example in the area of labour economics is the strong positive relationship between income and education. In this book, we focus on the case in which both responses are binary in nature. A bivariate binary logistic model with correlated random effects may be used to analyse a pair of repeated binary outcomes.

SABRE may be used to fit both of these generalizations. In Sub-section 4.5.2, we use SABRE to apply the ordinal logistic random effects model to the teenage drinking data. In Sub-section 4.5.3, we show how SABRE may be used to fit the bivariate binary logistic model with correlated random effects to paired response data from a linguistic study.

4.5.1. Model Fitting in SABRE:
Commands to Fit a Binary Logistic Model

The data for this example came from the study described in Section 5.2. The response variable is 'smoking' which has two possible values: '1' for smokers, and '0' for non-smokers. The dataset also provides demographic, social and health variables. SABRE can fit standard and random effects logistic models to data. The data structure must be appropriate for the model being fitted. The data file must be prepared and organised with variables in columns and cases as rows. In the case of longitudinal data or repeated measures, the records for each case must be on consecutive lines and with a case identifier which is usually the first variable in the dataset. For example, the first 11 lines and first 11 variables (columns) of data from the teenage smoking study are shown below:

```
Case-id  v1 v2 v3 v4 v5    v6      v7    v8 v9 v10
136099.0  4  2  2  3  2    .00    2.00    2  2  3
136099.0  6  2  2  2  2    .00    2.00    2  4  2
136101.0  4  2  2  1  2   1.00    1.00    1  3  2
136101.0  6  2  3  2  3   1.00    1.00    1  3  3
136105.0  5  2  3  2  2    .00    2.00    2  2  2
136105.0  7  2  3  2  2    .00    2.00    1  4  3
136106.0  5  2  1  2  2   1.00    2.00    1  3  3
136106.0  7  2  2  2  2   1.00    2.00    1  3  3
136107.0  4  2  2  3  2    .00    2.00    2  2  3
136107.0  6  2  1  3  2    .00    2.00    2  4  3
```

The SABRE commandfile used to read the data into SABRE and to fit binary logistic model to the data is given below.

```
data ID SMOK1 TIME SEX AGE CHOOSEAT TYPWGHT FRENSMOK PARTNER and
OPPSEX WYMONEY WYFAMILY ATLEAST1 DRINKS
read smok31.dat
yvar smok1
fac age fage
fac sex fsex
fac chooseat fchooseat
fac typwght ftypwght
fac frensmok ffrensmok
fac partner fpartner
fac oppsex foppsex
fac wymoney fwymoney
fac wyfamily fwyfamily
fac atleast1 fatleast1
fac drinks fdrinks
c
c pooled x-sectional logistic analysis
c
constant cons
lfit cons fsex fage fchooseat ftypwght ffrensmok fpartner and
foppsex fwymoney fwyfamily fatleast1 fdrinks
dis m
dis e
c
c logistic random effects model with mover/stayer
c
endpoints both
fit cons fsex fage fchooseat ftypwght ffrensmok fpartner and
foppsex fwymoney fwyfamily fatleast1 fdrinks
dis m
dis e
stop
```

The case identifier is the variable (column) case-id, age, sex and booze are the variables v1, v2 and v3 respectively and so on. The case identifier can be in any column but this must be declared to let SABRE know where to find it. The following output from SABRE shows the results from fitting two models: (i) a standard logistic model; (ii) a logistic model which incorporates both random effects and endpoints (mover/stayer).

The variables are declared using the data command and the data file smok31.dat is read using the read command. The response variable is smok1 and the categorical variables are declared with the fac statement. Notice that the SABRE command to fit a standard logistic model is lfit. To fit a random effects model with mover/stayer we use endpoints both and use the fit command.

The output from running the above SABRE commands is shown below. Note that, with older versions of SABRE (as below), the deviance of a fit was the default statistic displayed in the output whereas in later versions, including the latest version (version 6, see next example in Sub-section 4.5.2) the log-likelihood is displayed. The deviance is then -2*log-likelihood which is calculated by the user after the model has been fitted.

```
data ID SMOK1 TIME SEX AGE CHOOSEAT TYPWGHT FRENSMOK PARTNER and
OPPSEX WYMONEY WYFAMILY ATLEAST1 DRINKS
read smok31.dat

    1238 observations in dataset


c
c pooled x-sectional logistic analysis
c
lfit cons fsex fage fchooseat ftypwght ffrensmok fpartner and
foppsex fwymoney fwyfamily fatleast1 fdrinks
```

Iteration	Deviance	Reduction
1	1716.2324	
2	1212.0616	504.2
3	1166.2254	45.84
4	1162.9328	3.293
5	1162.9041	0.2870E-01
6	1162.9041	0.2796E-05

```
dis m   {this command displays the model fitted

    X-vars          Y-var
    ────────────────────────
    int             smok1
    fsex
    fage
    fchoos
    ftypwg
    ffrens
    fpartn
    foppse
    fwymon
    fwyfam
    fatlea
    fdrink

    Model type: standard binary logistic

    Number of observations      =    1238

    X-vars df          =    17

    Deviance           =    1162.9041    on  1221 residual degrees of
freedom

dis e   {this command displays the result of a fit e.g. parameter estimates
        {and standard errors
```

Parameter	Estimate	S. Error
int	0.23197	0.30529
fsex (1)	0.00000E+00	ALIASED [I]
fsex (2)	0.25395	0.16508
fage (1)	0.00000E+00	ALIASED [I]
fage (2)	0.50389	0.22861
fage (3)	0.29419	0.18559
fage (4)	0.34230	0.23457
fchoos(1)	0.00000E+00	ALIASED [I]
fchoos(2)	-0.65454	0.23381
fchoos(3)	-0.92736	0.27988
ftypwg(1)	0.00000E+00	ALIASED [I]
ftypwg(2)	-0.37850	0.15397
ffrens(1)	0.00000E+00	ALIASED [I]
ffrens(2)	-1.4973	0.16978
fpartn(1)	0.00000E+00	ALIASED [I]
fpartn(2)	-0.25711	0.15002
foppse(1)	0.00000E+00	ALIASED [I]
foppse(2)	-0.45041	0.25934
fwymon(1)	0.00000E+00	ALIASED [I]
fwymon(2)	0.19230	0.18963
fwymon(3)	0.62231	0.19586
fwyfam(1)	0.00000E+00	ALIASED [I]
fwyfam(2)	0.15506	0.18652
fwyfam(3)	0.21287	0.18179
fatlea(1)	0.00000E+00	ALIASED [I]
fatlea(2)	-0.48252	0.14972
fdrink(1)	0.00000E+00	ALIASED [I]
fdrink(2)	-1.2590	0.20750

```
c
c logistic random effects model with mover/stayer
c
endpoints both
fit cons fsex fage fchooseat ftypwght ffrensmok fpartner and
foppsex fwymoney fwyfamily fatleast1 fdrinks
```

Initial Logistic Fit:

Iteration	Deviance	Reduction
1	1716.2324	
2	1212.0616	504.2
3	1166.2254	45.84
4	1162.9328	3.293
5	1162.9041	0.2870E-01
6	1162.9041	0.2796E-05

Iteration	Deviance	Step length	End-points 0	1	Orthogonality criterion
1	1127.0189	1.0000	free	free	11.596
2	1089.0689	1.0000	free	free	4.8487
3	1085.3471	1.0000	free	free	11.310
4	1084.8514	1.0000	free	free	3.3200
5	1084.7633	1.0000	free	free	8.1638
6	1084.7373	1.0000	free	free	3.0955
7	1084.7239	1.0000	free	free	30.169
8	1084.7238	1.0000	free	free	

```
dis m

    X-vars      Y-var       Case-var
    int         smok1       id
    fsex
    fage
    fchoos
    ftypwg
    ffrens
    fpartn
    foppse
    fwymon
    fwyfam
    fatlea
    fdrink

    Model type: standard binary logistic-normal mixture with end-points

    Number of observations    =    1238
    Number of cases           =     619

    X-vars df        =    17
    Scale df         =     1
    End-point df     =     2

    Deviance         =    1084.7238    on   1218 residual degrees of freedom

dis e
```

Parameter	Estimate	S. Error		PROBABILITY
int	1.1833	0.51869		
fsex (1)	0.00000E+00	ALIASED [I]		
fsex (2)	0.25192	0.31571		
fage (1)	0.00000E+00	ALIASED [I]		
fage (2)	1.0028	0.35842		
fage (3)	0.74908	0.27430		
fage (4)	0.84515	0.38647		
fchoos(1)	0.00000E+00	ALIASED [I]		
fchoos(2)	-0.75077	0.39490		
fchoos(3)	-1.4448	0.46981		
ftypwg(1)	0.00000E+00	ALIASED [I]		
ftypwg(2)	-0.62831	0.25880		
ffrens(1)	0.00000E+00	ALIASED [I]		
ffrens(2)	-2.1857	0.28256		
fpartn(1)	0.00000E+00	ALIASED [I]		
fpartn(2)	-0.16125	0.25565		
foppse(1)	0.00000E+00	ALIASED [I]		
foppse(2)	-0.53691	0.41044		
fwymon(1)	0.00000E+00	ALIASED [I]		
fwymon(2)	0.13174	0.29410		
fwymon(3)	0.70641	0.31470		
fwyfam(1)	0.00000E+00	ALIASED [I]		
fwyfam(2)	0.51968	0.32382		
fwyfam(3)	0.43962	0.29114		
fatlea(1)	0.00000E+00	ALIASED [I]		
fatlea(2)	-0.70763	0.27087		
fdrink(1)	0.00000E+00	ALIASED [I]		
fdrink(2)	-1.8616	0.33006		
scale	0.68772	0.69407		
end-point 0	0.57695	0.16457		0.36027
end-point 1	0.24489E-01	0.21090E-01		0.15292E-01

```
stop
```

These results will be interpreted in Section 5.2.1.

4.5.2. Model Fitting in SABRE:
Commands to Fit an Ordinal Logistic Model

The following sample of SABRE commands relates to the teenage drinking example (Section 5.3) which has four possible outcomes: non-drinkers, low drinkers, medium drinkers and heavy drinkers. These ordered categories are based on the numbers of units of alcohol that the adolescent respondents were reported to have drunk (Sub-section 5.3.1.3).

```
c create output file for modelling teenage drinking

out alcohol3.txt

c model fitting for teenage alcohol
c
c yvar is ordinal drinking habit
c
c ==1 don't drink
c ==2 low drinker  (up to 7 units)
c ==3 medium drinker (8-20 units)
c ==4 heavy drinker   (21 plus units)

data id age sex booz howfit parknow smoke atleast &
frensmok maininf

read alcohol.dat

caseid id
fac sex fsex
fac age fage
fac howfit fith
fac parknow par
fac smoke smok
fac atleast at
fac frensmok best
fac maininf info

yvar booz

c fit the ordinal model

ordered y

c fit the null model

fit
dis m

c add each explanatory variable to the model separately
```

```
fit fsex
dis m

fit fage
dis m

fit fith
dis m

fit par
dis m

fit smok
dis m

c and so on...
```

The difference between this SABRE command file and the previous one is the way in which the model to be fitted is declared. In this latter example, the response variable takes values 1, 2, 3 or 4. After it is declared through the command `yvar booz`, another command is issued to tell SABRE this is an ordinal response variable: `ordered y`. The variable selection and model fitting then follow a similar pattern. We compare the deviance from each model fitted with the null model (i.e. deviance of null model - deviance of the new model). As we shall see in more detail in Sub-section 5.3.1, age makes the largest contribution towards explaining the variation in drinking, so age is selected to enter the model first. We add the remaining significant explanatory variables separately to the model which includes age, as follows:

```
c
c add age
c
fit fage
dis m

c
c add each remaining explanatory variable in turn, having controlled for
c age
c
fit fage fsex
dis m
dis e

fit fage par
dis m
dis e

fit fage smok
dis m
dis e

and so on ...
```

Subsequently, we compare the deviance of each new model with that of the model including age only (i.e. deviance of model with age - deviance of new model). We repeat the above process no variables remain significant at the 5% level.

For the interpretation of the results, see Sub-section 5.3.1.

4.5.3. Model Fitting in SABRE:
Commands to Fit Bivariate Binary Logistic Model

In this study, the sample of participants was grouped by gender, age and ethnicity. They were asked to listen to a group of speakers and then guess the speaker's ethnicity and locality they came from (see Sub-section 5.4.1). For each of the ethnicity and location variables, the binary response of 'guessed correctly' (1) and 'guessed incorrectly' (0) was recorded. In other words, the study observed two binary responses in parallel. This type of data is referred to as a bivariate binary response. SABRE can handle bivariate and trivariate response data. Before fitting models to the data in SABRE, we must carry out some data preparation.

To organise an appropriate data structure for this type of model, consider a bivariate dataset as being two univariate datasets put together in order to fit two univariate models simultaneously (and thereby allowing us to take into account the correlation between the two responses). Each half of the bivariate dataset has a `yvar` just as it would for a univariate model. The distribution of the `yvar` for the first response is not necessarily the same as that for the second response. For example, the first response could be binary (0,1) and associated with a logit model, but the second response could be continuous (any real value) and associated with a linear model. These two responses are joined together (stacked on top of one another in the dataset) and become the single response variable `yvar`. The variable `rvar` indicates which half of the dataset each observation comes from and takes the value 1 in the first half of the dataset (referring to the first response variable) and 2 in the second half of the dataset (referring to the second response variable). The indicator variables `r1` and `r2` are then derived from `rvar`: `r1 = 1 if rvar = 1`, `r1 = 0 if rvar = 2`; `r2 = 0 if rvar = 1`, `r2 = 1 if rvar = 2`. So, in a bivariate dataset with two binary response variables, this part of the data would look like:

yvar	rvar	r1	r2
0	1	1	0
0	1	1	0
1	1	1	0
0	1	1	0
.	.	.	.
.	.	.	.
.	.	.	.
1	2	0	1
0	2	0	1
1	2	0	1
0	2	0	1
.	.	.	.
.	.	.	.
.	.	.	.

Explanatory variables are included in the model as interaction terms with r1 and/or r2. These interaction terms can be created in SABRE using the transform command. For example, to fit the sex effect in the model, we first create the variable r1_stim_sex using the transform command trans r1_stim_sex r1 * stimulus_sex, and use transform in a similar manner for r2 and then include the variables r1_stim_sex and r1_stim_sex in the model. A sample of SABRE commands used to fit bivariate binary logistic model follows:

```
data ij r listener_code listener_group listener_ethnicity &
   listener_sex stimulus_number stimulus_sex stimulus_network &
   ethnicity_reply ethnicity_score location_reply location_score
   y & r1 r2 stim_net1 stim_net2 stim_net3 stim_net4 stim_net5

read london_biv_stimulus.dat

case stimulus_number    {declaring stimulus_number as the random
                        {effect
yvar y                  {declaring y as the response variable
model b                 {declaring the model to be bivariate
corr n                  {assuming independence between the two
                        {binary responses
rvar r                  {declaring r as pointer for y (see above)

constant first=r1 second=r2

c create interaction terms between r1, r2
c and the explanatory variables
trans r1_stim_sex r1 * stimulus_sex
trans r1_stim_net3 r1 * stim_net3
trans r1_stim_net4 r1 * stim_net4
trans r1_stim_net5 r1 * stim_net5
trans r2_stim_sex r2 * stimulus_sex
trans r2_stim_net3 r2 * stim_net3
trans r2_stim_net4 r2 * stim_net4
trans r2_stim_net5 r2 * stim_net5
nvar 5      {specifying the number of variables including r1/r2
            {per response in the linear predictor

c fit the standard logistic model

lfit r1 r1_stim_sex r1_stim_net3 r1_stim_net4 r1_stim_net5 &
     r2 r2_stim_sex r2_stim_net3 r2_stim_net4 r2_stim_net5

dis m

quad a      {using adaptive quadrature method for the random
            {effects model
```

```
nvar 5         {specifying the number of variables including r1/r2
               {per response in the linear predictor
c
c fit a random effects model
c
fit r1 r1_stim_sex r1_stim_net3 r1_stim_net4 r1_stim_net5 &
    r2 r2_stim_sex r2_stim_net3 r2_stim_net4 r2_stim_net5

dis m

corr y         {assume the two binary outcomes are correlated
nvar 5
c
c fit a random effects model
c
fit r1 r1_stim_sex r1_stim_net3 r1_stim_net4 r1_stim_net5 &
    r2 r2_stim_sex r2_stim_net3 r2_stim_net4 r2_stim_net5
dis m

dis e

stop
```

The output from running the above SABRE commands is shown below. For the interpretation of the results, see Sub-section 5.4.1.

```
read london_biv_stimulus.dat

     1024 observations in dataset

c fit the standard logistic model

lfit r1 r1_stim_sex r1_stim_net3 r1_stim_net4 r1_stim_net5 &
    r2 r2_stim_sex r2_stim_net3 r2_stim_net4 r2_stim_net5

dis m

    Log likelihood =      -578.73155        on      1014 residual
degrees of freedom

dis e

        Parameter              Estimate        Std. Err.
        ─────────────────────────────────────────────────
        r1                     0.46365         0.41702
        r1_stim_sex            0.92265         0.22114
```

```
            r1_stim_net3        -0.65937           0.43257
            r1_stim_net4        -2.6672            0.50277
            r1_stim_net5        -2.3641            0.40028
            r2                  -0.36821           0.38990
            r2_stim_sex         -0.38556           0.24517
            r2_stim_net3         1.7524            0.39400
            r2_stim_net4         2.4714            0.51030
            r2_stim_net5         2.3767            0.37177

quad a      {using adaptive quadrature method for the random
             {effects model
nvar 5      {specifying the number of variables including r1/r2
             per response in the linear predictor
c fit a random effects model

fit r1 r1_stim_sex r1_stim_net3 r1_stim_net4 r1_stim_net5 &
    r2 r2_stim_sex r2_stim_net3 r2_stim_net4 r2_stim_net5

dis m

    Log likelihood =      -551.74567        on      1012 residual
degrees of freedom

dis e

            Parameter           Estimate           Std. Err.

            r1                   0.43960           1.1169
            r1_stim_sex          0.97903           0.62281
            r1_stim_net3        -0.74451           1.1736
            r1_stim_net4        -2.7306            1.3122
            r1_stim_net5        -2.4258            1.0546
            r2                  -0.33928           0.52206
            r2_stim_sex         -0.42213           0.31741
            r2_stim_net3         1.7777            0.53222
            r2_stim_net4         2.4977            0.64949
            r2_stim_net5         2.4588            0.50038
            scale1               0.85459           0.21647
            scale2               0.28126           0.16413

   corr y   {assume the two binary outcomes are correlated
   nvar 5

   c fit an independent random effects model

   fit r1 r1_stim_sex r1_stim_net3 r1_stim_net4 r1_stim_net5 &
       r2 r2_stim_sex r2_stim_net3 r2_stim_net4 r2_stim_net5
dis m
```

```
     Log likelihood =      -551.67416        on       1011 residual
degrees of freedom

dis e
```

Parameter	Estimate	Std. Err.
r1	0.43896	1.1192
r1_stim_sex	0.97960	0.62408
r1_stim_net3	-0.74539	1.1759
r1_stim_net4	-2.7305	1.3149
r1_stim_net5	-2.4243	1.0567
r2	-0.34777	0.52935
r2_stim_sex	-0.41376	0.32168
r2_stim_net3	1.7740	0.53982
r2_stim_net4	2.4982	0.65703
r2_stim_net5	2.4581	0.50654
scale1	0.85665	0.21712
scale2	0.28984	0.16688
corr	0.19031	0.48867

```
stop
```

4.6. Using SABRE with Commercial Packages

SABRE is available as a plug-in for the commercial package Stata (http://www.lancs.ac.uk/staff/cpajp/SABRE/ SABREStatause_intro.html). A SABREStata coursebook with associated example .do files, data files and coursebook exercises are available via links in the left-hand menu.

SABRE is also available as an R library. Its use is described in the SABRER coursebook which can be downloaded via the link in the left-hand menu. http://www.lancs.ac.uk/staff/cpajp/SABRE/SABRERuse_intro.html

Chapter 5

EXAMPLES OF SABRE APPLICATION

5.1. INTRODUCTION

In the previous chapters, we discussed and demonstrated the substantive reasons for ensuring a proper analytical framework. Recall from Chapter 1 that substantive issues relate to the dynamics of processes. In the context of human behaviour, most processes are dynamic i.e. temporal dependencies or changes over time influence the process outcome from one point in time to another. The main issues considered in this book were the omitted variables or heterogeneity effect, the feedback effect and past behaviour and multicollinearity. These issues are prevalent in data regardless of whether the data were obtained cross-sectionally or longitudinally. An understanding of the issues related to the dynamics of a process necessitates extra flexibility in the analysis and informs interpretation of the results e.g. the analysis described in Section 3.6.2. As these issues have been explicitly discussed in previous chapters, the issues are implied through the adopted methodology in the example analyses in this chapter. We proceed to demonstrate the applications of SABRE described in the previous chapter using secondary data sources. We conduct longitudinal analyses of univariate binary teenage smoking habit data, multinomial (ordinal) teenage alcohol consumption habit data, and bivariate binary paired outcomes from a socio-linguistic study.

The applications are presented as fully worked examples rather than simply as exercises in SABRE data entry and output. In this way, SABRE input and output are an integral part of the presentation. The reader interested in the SABRE commands used to fit the various models in this chapter could refer back to Chapter 4, in particular Sub-sections 4.4.1, 4.4.2 and 4.4.3.

5.2. EXAMPLE 1: UNIVARIATE BINARY RESPONSE

5.2.1. Teenage Smoking

5.2.1.1. Background

Teenage smoking is a decision process which is influenced by social processes. In studying a decision to smoke or not, we must therefore consider the issues of human behaviour discussed thus far (also see [29, 30]). The literature on smoking reports a large number of variables to be associated with teenage smoking. For example, smoking has been associated with demographic, social, environmental, economic, emotional and psychological variables [120-126]. Specifically, smoking behaviour has been associated with the psychosocial effect of wishing to belong to a peer social group [127], with self-esteem and parental smoking behaviour [128], and with the psychological process of risk assessment and risk-taking [129-131]. Smoking behaviour has also been linked to the family environment, which in turn affects psychological well-being and may cause problems with adjustment and behaviour, perceived academic performance and school conduct [132, 133]. Furthermore, the feedback effect of smoking has been reported as the subjective effect of smoking e.g. feelings of higher self-esteem and being in control [128, 134], and **a perceived 'benefit' effect as** utilised in risk models [129, 130]. How the explanatory variables are related with each other will have an impact on the final results. This is referred to as multicollinearity (see Subsection 1.2.2).

The major issues which arise when dealing with survey type studies, such as past behaviour and omitted variables, were discussed in detail in Chapters 2 and 3. For example, omitted characteristics, such as resilience, could lead to spurious relationships between the observed characteristics and the outcome variable. A consequence of such a relationship may be an overestimation of the effects of explanatory variables on smoking. In this context, within the literature, residual heterogeneity due to omitted variables is commonly referred to as heterogeneity. In this chapter, the terms residual heterogeneity, omitted variables and heterogeneity are used interchangeably to refer to inherent individual-specific variability (e.g. personality, resilience). Conventional statistical analysis such as standard regression models subsume the individual-specific heterogeneity into the structural error term, thus violating the independence assumption and leading to a well-known specification error [14, 87].

A past behaviour effect exists when the experience of a particular outcome itself changes the probability of experiencing that event on subsequent occasions. It is also important to have measures of past behaviour on smoking and on the explanatory variables in order to gain some insight into the direction of causality e.g. the confidence-smoking relationship. For example, Murphy et al. [128] reported low self-esteem among the female group who indicated an intention to smoke. This means the assertion that more confident individuals are more likely to be smokers [135] may become untenable, as it is likely that the individuals had lower self-esteem prior to taking up smoking. It is not surprising that researchers [136, 137], applying a cross-sectional statistical technique to longitudinal data, reported a high correlation between smoking status in adolescence and that outcome in adulthood - as a cessation will often be accompanied by feelings of unease and anxiety [132, 138].

Most studies of teenage smoking have relied on cross-sectional observational or survey questionnaire data. Although multicollinearity can be addressed with cross-sectional data, to address the omitted variables and past behaviour effects, longitudinal data are required. However, inappropriate analytical methods that do not utilise fully the longitudinal nature of data, e.g. by not accounting for heterogeneity, will lead to erroneus results and misleading conclusions e.g. see [136, 137, 139-143]. One study [142] had accounted for the past behaviour effect but this had been achieved within a cross-sectional analytical framework. The possibility exists that the past behaviour effect owes its significance to a well-known misspecification error where the included explanatory variable (in this case past behaviour), through omitted variables, may be correlated with the structural error, see Chapter 3.

Analysis of teenage smoking has been reported elsewhere in full [29, 30, 144-146]. As mentioned above, in this section we demonstrate the application of a longitudinal statistical modelling approach using SABRE to the two-time point smoking data from a health-related behaviour survey.

5.2.1.2. Data

In 1992, 60 secondary schools in the former Yorkshire Regional Health Authority geographical boundary (UK) agreed to take part in a health behaviour-related survey to be repeated every two years. Years 9 and 11 (age range 11-16 years) in these schools were surveyed using a health-related behaviour questionnaire [147]. These surveys were anonymous and were not linked. This limitation restricted the analysis to comparative cross-sectional analyses of change in proportion of outcomes of interest. The 1994 survey was modified to include a form to be filled in by those who were in their final school year (16+ year olds). The form merely invited the pupils to indicate their interest to participate in a follow-up survey in two years time and if so to fill in their contact details. Organisational changes within the National Health Service (NHS) during 1994 saw the abolition of the Regional Health Authorities in England and by 1996 the Yorkshire Regional Health Authority had ceased to exist. However, the survey was conducted as planned and 627 young adults were traced and re-interviewed using the same questionnaire instrument with slight modifications to some questions to suit the 18+ age category.

The questionnaire covered topics related to the attitudes and behaviour of the pupils with regard to health e.g. physical exercise and out-of-school activities, nutrition, social contacts, dealing with problems, attitudes to and the use of drugs (including smoking and drinking). For the purpose of this chapter, we will use SABRE to test the cross-sectional model reported elsewhere [29] which is shown in Tables 5.1. The outcome variable 'smoking' is a binary variable which takes the value '0' if a non-smoker (those who claimed they have never smoked or have given up smoking) and the value '1' if a smoker (those who claimed they smoked either regularly or occasionally).

The descriptive analyses shown in Tables 5.2(b-c) suggest that out of the 627 subjects there were 619 valid cases; 62.5% were female and 37.5% were male; 22% of the 1994 sample were smokers the proportion of which increased to 33% in 1996. However, over the two year period, there was no noticeable change in the proportion of smokers by gender. Over this period, there were movements in the smoking status as follows (Table 5.2c): 61% remained non-smokers, 17% remained smokers, 17% were non-smokers in 1994 but smokers in 1996, and 5% were smokers in 1994 but non-smokers in 1996.

This dataset provides only two time observations **on a young adult's health**-related behaviour. More linked observations on the individuals prior to 1994 and post-1996 are essential to enable us to unravel some of the complexities of interactions between life processes and whatever impact they may have on smoking status over time. However, even with two time observations per individual, we can illustrate the added value from a statistical modelling perspective.

Table 5.1. Results of fitting binary logistic model of smoking (one explanatory variable at a time); N=1238

Explanatory Variables	Chi-sq	p
Gender	4.16	0.0244
Age	26.92	0.0000
At least one family member smokes	40.10	0.0000
Drinks	91.16	0.0000
Best friend smokes	172.42	0.0000
Consider health when choosing food	9.15	0.0124
Happy with weight	10.76	0.0006
Have a partner	29.85	0.0000
At ease with opposite sex	13.56	0.0001
Worry about money	55.40	0.0000
Worry about family problems	14.81	0.0003

Table 5.1a. Smoking status by gender in 1994

1994		Sex		Total
Freqs (Col %s)		Male	Female	
Smoker	No	188 (81.0%)	296 (76.5%)	484 (78.2%)
	Yes	44 (19.0%)	91 (23.5%)	135 (21.8%)
Total		232 (100%)	387 (100%)	619 (100%)

Table 5.1b. Smoking status by gender in 1996

1996		Sex		Total
Freqs (Col %s)		Male	Female	
Smoker	No	164 (70.4%)	248 (64.2%)	412 (66.6%)
	Yes	69 (29.6%)	138 (35.8%)	207 (33.4%)
Total		233 (100%)	386 (100%)	619 (100%)

Table 5.1c. Smoking status in 1994 by smoking status in 1996

		Smoker 1996		Total
Freqs (Col %s)		No	Yes	
Smoker 1994	No	380 (92.2%)	104 (50.2%)	484 (78.2 %)
	Yes	32 (7.8%)	103 (49.8%)	135 (21.8%)
Total		412 (100%)	207 (100%)	619 (100%)

5.2.1.3. Statistical Analysis Using SABRE

The outcome variable is a binary variable: '0' for non-smoker; '1' for smoker. With a binary response variable and many explanatory variables, the common statistical approach is to fit the standard logistic regression model to the data (as we did in Section 2.4). This model was fitted to the data. This led to the variables shown in Table 5.1 being selected in the cross-sectional analysis [29]. For comparison purposes, we fit the longitudinal model, described in Chapters 3 and 4 using SABRE, to the data using only the variables shown in Table 5.1 . The statistical modelling approach we have adopted allows control for secondary variables when testing a primary variable of interest. For example, to investigate the effect of the variable 'worry about money' on smoking, variables such as age, sex, happy with weight, whether drinks, and so on, are controlled for; in other words, are included in themodel first before the variable 'worry about money' is added to the model. However, of particular concern is the longitudinal nature of the data set. The standard logistic regression is essentially a cross-sectional model and fitting such a model to longitudinal data will lead to a well-known specification error and misleading results [12]. The model applied in this section is the logistic-normal random effects model [13, 148, 149] which allows for the possibility that substantial variation between respondents will be due to the heterogeneity which was discussed in Chapter 1.. This model incorporates a normal mixing distribution to account for the possibility of residual heterogeneity (scale parameter ω - Tables 5.4 and 5.5) (see Appendix VII). SABRE can fit such models to data. Another important issue that is often neglected is that some individuals will never (or will have a very low probability of) change, i.e. will always (or almost always) be a smoker or will never smoke. These individuals are referred to as 'stayers'. SABRE provides the additional flexibility of incorporating 'stayers' into the model by supplementing the normal mixing distribution with mass-points at plus orminus infinity (+/- ∞) (see Appendix VII). Three models were fitted in SABRE: (i) ordinary logistic regression model (Table 5.3), (ii) a logistic-normal random effects model assuming no stayers (Table 5.4), and (iii) a logistic-normal random effects model with stayers (Table 5.5). With only two timepoints, it is not practical for us to control for past behaviour in this case, though it is possible to do so in SABRE. A sample of the SABRE command file used to produce Tables 5.3-5.5 is provided in Sub-section 4.5.1. The interested reader is also referred to Appendix X for a complete list of SABRE commands.

Table 5.3. Results from pooled cross-sectional analysis; N=1,238 (Deviance=1162.9)

Explanatory Variables	p.e.	s.e.	χ^2	p
Gender			2.4	0.12
Male	0.00			
Female	0.25	0.17		
Age			5.6	0.13
15 and under	0.00			
16 years	0.50	0.23		
17 years	0.29	0.19		
18 and over	0.34	0.23		
At least one family member smokes			10.4	0.001
No	0.00			
Yes	0.48	0.15		
Drinks			42.9	0.0000
No	0.00			
Yes	1.26	0.21		
Best friend smokes			88	0.0000
No	0.00			
Yes	1.49	0.17		
Consider health when choosing food			11.2	0.004
Never	0.00			
Sometimes	-0.66	0.23		
Always	-0.93	0.28		

Table 5.3. – (Continued)

	p.e.	s.e.	χ²	p
Happy with weight			9	0.003
Put on/lose	0.00			
Happy	-0.38	0.15		
Have a partner			2.9	0.09
No	0.00			
Yes	0.26	0.15		
At ease with opposite sex			3.2	0.07
No	0.00			
Yes	0.45	0.25		
Worry about money			11.2	0.004
Never	0.00			
A little	0.19	0.19		
A lot	0.62	0.19		
Worry about family problems			1.5	0.47
Never	0.00			
A little	0.16	0.19		
A lot	0.21	0.18		

Table 5.4. Results from longitudinal analysis without stayers; N=619 Deviance=1091.26)

Explanatory Variables	p.e.	s.e.	χ²	p
Gender			1.8	0.1800
Male	0.00			
Female	0.43	0.32		
Age			10.5	0.0100
15 and under	0.00			
16 years	0.99	0.39		
17 years	0.74	0.28		
18 and over	0.86	0.41		
At least one family member smokes			7.4	0.0060
No	0.00			
Yes	0.76	0.28		
Drinks			39	0.0000
No	0.00			
Yes	1.99	0.37		
Best friend smokes			76	0.0000
No	0.00			
Yes	2.29	0.31		
Consider health when choosing food			6.9	0.0300
Never	0.00			
Sometimes	-0.72	0.41		
Always	-1.28	0.49		
Happy with weight			5.7	0.0200
Put on/lose	0.00			
Happy	-0.63	0.27		
Have a partner			1.3	0.2500
No	0.00			
Yes	0.29	0.26		
At ease with opposite sex			2.1	>>0.1
Yes	0.00			
No	-0.59	0.41		
Worry about money			5.7	0.0500
Never	0.00			
Explanatory Variables	p.e.	s.e.	χ²	P
A little	0.12	0.31		
A lot	0.72	0.33		
Worry about family problems			2.82	0.2500
Never	0.00			
A little	0.42	0.32		
A lot	0.47	0.31		
Scale (ω)	2.38	0.31		

Table 5.5. Results from longitudinal analysis with stayers; N=619 (Deviance=1084.72)

Explanatory Variables	p.e.	s.e.	χ^2	p
Gender			0.6	0.44
Male	0.00	0.32		
Female	0.25			
Age			12	0.007
15 and under	0.00			
16 years	1.00	0.36		
17 years	0.75	0.27		
18 and over	0.85	0.39		
At least one family member smokes			7.2	0.007
No	0.00			
Yes	0.71	0.27		
Drinks			39	0.0000
No	0.00			
Yes	1.86	0.33		
Best friend smokes			80.5	0.0000
No	0.00			
Yes	2.19	0.28		
Consider health when choosing food			10.1	0.007
Never	0.00			
Sometimes	-0.75	0.39		
Always	-1.45	0.47		
Happy with weight			6.2	0.01
Put on/lose	0.00			
Happy	-0.63	0.26		
Have a partner			0.4	0.53
No	0.00			
Yes	0.16	0.26		
At ease with opposite sex			1.7	0.19
No	0.00			
Yes	0.54	0.41		
Worry about money			5.8	0.05
Never	0.00			
A little	0.13	0.29		
A lot	0.71	0.31		
Worry about family problems			3.4	0.18
Never	0.00			
A little	0.52	0.32		
A lot	0.44	0.29		
Scale (ω)	0.69	0.69		
			PROBABILITY	
ψ_0 (end-point0)	0.58	0.16	0.36	
ψ_1 (end-point1)	0.02	0.02	0.01	

5.2.1.4. Interpretation of Results

Tables 5.3-5.5 show the results from fitting the three models: (i) a standard conventional logistic model to the pooled data from 1994 and 1996 (Table 5.3), (ii) a logistic-normal random effects model assuming no stayers (Table 5.4) and (iii) a logistic-normal random effects model with stayers (Table 5.5). The tables provide the list of variables and their categories, their parameter estimates and standard errors, chi-squared (χ^2) goodness of fit tests and their associated p-values. The statistical significance of a variable in the model is indicated by the χ^2 and its associated p-value. For this analysis, the significance level was set to 5% ($\alpha=0.05$). Thus, a χ^2 showing a p-value of less than or equal to 0.05 (e.g. <0.005, <0.0001) would indicate a statistically significant variable in the model. Positive estimates indicate likelihood of being a smoker compared with the reference category (usually the first category) e.g. 16 year old pupils are more likely to be smokers than those 15 and under. Similarly, negative estimates indicate likelihood of being a non-smoker e.g. those who claimed that their best friend did not smoke are less likely to be smoker (or more likely to be non-smoker) than those whose best friend was a smoker. As demonstrated in Chapter 6 and in Appendix II, the parameter estimates can be translated easily into odds ratios (ORs) and interpreted accordingly. However, in this section our main concern is the comparison of the parameter estimates and their standard errors from the cross-sectional model to those from the longitudinal model.

With the standard logistic regression model, the variables gender and 'worry about family problems' appear non-significant after controlling for other variables. Both variables were significant on their own at the 5% significance level. Similarly, age, which was highly significant on its own, is now only marginally significant after controlling for other variables. Out of the remaining variables, 'at ease with opposite sex' and 'have a partner' are also marginally significant (at the 10% level). All the other variables in the model appear to be significant at the 5% level.

In general, the results suggest that having non-smoking family members, not drinking, considering health when choosing food and not worrying about money problems appear to reduce the likelihood of being a smoker. Furthermore, for each parameter estimate, an odds ratio and 95% confidence interval can be calculated, as in Table 5.6.

Table 5.6. odds ratios (ORs) and 95% confidence intervals (C.I) for the variable 'best friend smokes'

	p.e.	s.e.	OR	Lower C.I band	Upper C.I band
From Table 5.3					
No	0.00		1.00		
Yes	1.49	0.17	4.47	3.20	6.23
From Table 5.4					
No	0.00		1.00		
Yes	2.29	0.31	9.88	5.42	18.04
From Table 5.5					
No	0.00		1.00		
Yes	2.19	0.28	8.90	5.11	15.50

The interpretation of the results is informed by comparing Tables 5.4 and 5.5. In particular, the important information is the change in the scale parameter and the probability of being a stayer. The change in deviance from the standard logistic model to the logistic-normal random effects model without stayers is highly significant (1162.9 – 1091.3 = 71.6 on 1 d.f.), as is the estimate of the scale parameter (ω) (Table 5.4), indicating that there is substantial residual heterogeneity due to omitted variables. The results suggest that ignoring heterogeneity may lead to underestimation. The change in deviance from the random effects model without stayers to the random effects model with stayers is significant at the 5% level (1091.3 – 1084.7 = 6.6 on 2 d.f.), indicating that there is a significant proportion of stayers in the sample. Indeed, inspection of the estimate of endpoint parameter 0 (ψ_0) (Table 5.5) reveals a highly significant proportion of stayers in state 0; in other words, 36% of the pupils claimed both in 1994 and in 1996 that they had never smoked or had given up smoking (be it prior to 1994 or within the 1994-1996 project window). Endpoint parameter 1 (ψ_1) is not significant at the 5% level: only 1% of the pupils claimed that they had smoked either regularly or occasionally both in 1994 and in 1996. The scale parameter (ω) is no longer significant; in other words, the residual heterogeneity revealed by the previous model has been explained by the high proportion of non-smoking stayers in the current model.

Age is the only objective variable remaining in the models. The effects of the remaining variables are diminished. Furthermore, an examination of the parameter estimates and their standard errors suggests that the standard logistic model has underestimated the effects of these variables. For example, Table 5.6 shows the odds ratios with the corresponding 95% confidence intervals for the variable 'best friend smokes' in all three models. Based on the results of the two random effects models, it can be seen that the effect of 'best friend', though statistically significant, has been estimated with less precision, given the wider confidence intervals, compared to that derived from the standard model.

The change in the age effect from the standard logistic model to the logistic-normal model serves to demonstrate the complex inter-relationships in the data due to the presence of the subjective variables. The effects of the subjective variables are inflated, very likely due to their relationship with the outcome variable, smoking, through the omitted variables (see also [29]). The age effect may appear to be marginally significant in Table 5.3. However, when controlling for residual heterogeneity, in Tables 5.4 and 5.5, the age effect appears to be statistically significant.

The results, based on our sample, can be interpreted as follows: the likelihood of being a smoker appears to increase: with age; with exposure to smoking and drinking as measured by the variables 'at least one family member smokes', 'best friend smokes' and 'drinks'; with emotional dependence as measured by the variables 'happy with weight' and 'worry about money'. The likelihood of being a smoker seems to decrease with having a healthy attitude as measured by the variable 'consider health when choosing food'. The variable 'worry about money' is only marginally significant and the remaining variables are non-significant. Perhaps the most important aspect of these results is the statistically significant 'omitted variables' effects as estimated by the scale parameter ω.

5.2.1.5. Discussion

As discussed in Chapters 1, 2 and 3, the possibility of a past behaviour effect (e.g. state dependence and duration dependence) should not be discounted. It would have been preferable to follow up pupils from an earlier age before the uptake of smoking, and to collect observations on more than two time points, thereby allowing us to incorporate past behaviour, pathways to smoking/giving up smoking, and other dynamics of behaviour into the analysis. The model does not account for time-varying heterogeneity (such as the feel good factor). Some of these limitations, e.g. accounting for time-varying heterogeneity, may be overcome by adopting a pragmatic multi-method approach, e.g. see Sub-section 3.8.3.

However, the purpose of this example is to demonstrate the effects of omitted variables on the estimates of parameters in standard logistic and logistic-normal random effects models. The effects of omitted variables, if they exist, are to inflate the relationship between the outcome variable (smoking) and the explanatory variables by underestimating the standard errors [14, 87]. Indeed, the comparison of the results from the standard and random effects models (Tables 5.3, 5.4 and 5.5) suggests such overestimation due to the omitted variables. Almost a half of the explanatory variables that were reported as significant in the standard logistic regression model ceased to be significant in the random effects models. Furthermore, the standard model appeared to underestimate the standard errors. For example, the peer pressure effect (the variable 'best friend smokes') in itself may not be a direct and independent effect on smoking. In fact, this variable may owe its significance, at least in part, to an unobserved phenomenon or a latent variable such as a resilience factor [150] that influences teenage decision-making. Resilience in turn may be governed by personal characteristics and other social and environmental variables e.g. parental influence [151-153], and the media (e.g. [154]). This means that the act of being 'happy with weight' or 'worrying' may not directly increase the likelihood of being a smoker. Such variables appear to be highly correlated with the omitted variables, thereby acting as proxies for individual characteristics which had not been measured. Failure to address the substantive and analytical issues may lead to inconsistencies in results (e.g. as in [126, 155]) and misleading conclusions. These results support the earlier findings [29] that the relationship between smoking and self-esteem, confidence, stress levels, worrying about problems and money, health attitude and peer pressure could well be due to omitted variables.

For example, based on a review of the literature, Tyas [126] suggested that smoking is often used as a mechanism to cope with stress. The results from the random effects models, Tables 5.4 and 5.5, suggest that worrying about family problems and being at ease with the opposite sex are no longer significant, and worrying about money is significant at the 10% level. The calming effect of smoking is only reported by smokers and is related to the heightened effect of stress/anxiety and/or worrying on patterns of smoking in the population of smokers. The calming effect of smoking as a reason for smoking is not fully justified even when it is reported by the respondents themselves. Most of the studies reviewed by Tyas are cross-sectional and do not provide historical information on smoking. The calming effect of smoking could well be a feed-back effect, rather than a response to stress or worry, as a cessation of smoking will often be accompanied by feelings of unease and anxiety [132, 138]. This ambiguity in interpreting the results is further exacerbated by the subjective effect of smoking, e.g. feelings of higher self-esteem and being in control [128, 132]; and a perceived 'benefit' effect as utilised in risk models [129, 130] (see also Sub-section 5.3.1.5).

5.2.1.6. Summary

In this example, we have demonstrated that, through the appropriate application of statistical modelling, as in most social processes, there will be substantial residual heterogeneity in data due to omitted variables. Therefore, caution must be exercised in interpreting results. For example, using structural equation modelling, Flay et al. [156] suggested that the 'best friend' effect on adolescent initiation into smoking is a direct effect, whilst the analyses presented here suggest that at least some of the variation explained by the 'best friend' effect may well be due to its correlation with the omitted variables. We need to take a holistic approach to understanding what factors govern the dynamic psycho-social and individual characteristics that themselves **influence young people's** decision-making

5.3. EXAMPLE 2: MULTINOMIAL (ORDINAL) RESPONSE

5.3.1. Teenage Alcohol Drinking

5.3.1.1. Background

Alcohol has been associated with morbidity, including cancers and heart disease, and mortality [157, 158]. The literature links smoking with a drinking habit, and in turn, smoking and drinking are associated with young people's experimenting with and future use of illicit drugs [159-161]. In addition to smoking, individual characteristics, parental drinking patterns and socio-economic variables have also been used to predict drinking patterns, e.g. see [162-164]. However, the current knowledge is based on evidence from cross-sectional studies. But drinking, like smoking, is the outcome of a decision process. Processes are, by nature, dynamic.

As has been emphasised throughout this book, the issues of multicollinearity, residual heterogeneity and past behaviour must be addressed explicitly. Multicollinearity may be conceptualised as the relationship between observed explanatory variables masking the true effect of each explanatory variable on the response variable. For example, drinking has been associated with demographic, social, environmental, smoking and other drug use, TV advertising, economic, emotional and psychological (parental and peer pressure influence) variables [165-175]. Also, as described in the previous example, smoking behaviour, in turn, has been associated with psycho-social variables over and above demographic and socio-economic variables. How these explanatory variables are related with each other will have an impact on the final results (e.g. see [19], page 105).

By now, the reader should be familiar with the past behaviour effect and residual heterogeneity which have been discussed throughout this book and further described in the previous example. In these regards, teenage drinking behaviour is no different to teenage smoking behaviour.

Most studies of teenage drinking have relied on cross-sectional observational or survey questionnaire data. Although multicollinearity can be addressed with cross-sectional data, to address the issues of omitted variables and past behaviour effects, longitudinal data are required. However, even when a longitudinal study design is used, researchers have applied cross-sectional statistical techniques for data analysis or have used methods that do not utilise fully the longitudinal nature of the data (e.g see [162, 176-179]).

In this example, we demonstrate the application of a longitudinal statistical modelling approach to the two-time point drinking data from the health-related behaviour survey introduced in example 1 (see Section 5.2).

5.3.1.2. Data

Data on units of alcohol consumed, on drug use and on other explanatory variables from the Health Related Behaviour Questionnaire (see previous example) were used for this example. The outcome variable 'drinking' has four categories as follows: (1) 0 units (a non-drinker), (2) 1-7 units (a light drinker), (3) 8-20 units (a moderate drinker) and (4) 21 or more units (a heavy drinker) based upon the reported number of units consumed. The descriptive analyses shown in Tables 5.7(a-e) suggest that out of the 627 subjects there were 617 valid cases. For the purpose of this chapter, the relevant explanatory variables (see Table 5.9) were extracted from the data set. Tables 5.7 (a-b) show that 62.5% were female and 37.5% were male; 36% of the 1994 sample were non-drinkers, the proportion of which decreased to 21.6% in 1996. Tables 5.7 (a-b) also show that 7.8% of the males and 4.4% of females reported to be heavy drinkers in 1994, the proportion of which increased to 28.1% and 10.4% respectively. From 1994 to 1996, (Table 5.7e) over half of the non-drinkers had switched drinking status; 42% had remained non-drinkers, 27% had become light drinkers, 22% had become moderate drinkers and 9.5% had become heavy drinkers. Conversely, there were more drinkers in 1996: proportionally, those who drank in 1994 appear to drink more in 1996. For example, 43% of those who had classed themselves as light drinkers (up to 7 units) in 1994 were drinking 8-20 units in 1996, and 16% were heavy drinkers in 1996. This pattern can also be observed for the moderate and heavy drinking categories. As mentioned in Sub-section 5.3.1.1, smoking has been linked to drinking. We should therefore, remind ourselves of the dynamics of smoking status. Over this period, there were movements in the smoking status as follows (see Sub-section 5.2.1, Table 5.1c): 61% remained non-smokers, 17% remained smokers, 17% were non-smokers in 1994 but smokers in 1996, and 5% were smokers in 1994 but non-smokers in 1996.

Table 5.7. Some descriptive data analyses

a- Drinking status in 1994 by gender (column %s)

Drinking status	Sex Male	Female	Total
Don't drink	83(35.9%)	139(36.0%)	222(36.0%)
Light drinker	78(33.8%)	160(41.5%)	238(38.6%)
Moderate drinker	52(22.5%)	70(18.1)	122(19.8%)
Heavy drinker	18(7.8%)	17(4.4)	35(5.7%)
Total	231(37.5%)	386(62.5%)	617(100%)
Pearson Chi-sq	6.54	(p=0.09)	

b- Drinking status in 1996 by gender (column %s)

Drinks status	Sex Male	Female	Total
Don't drink	45(19.5%)	88(22.8%)	133(21.6%)
Light drinker	38(16.5%)	123(31.9%)	161(26.1%)
Moderate drinker	83(35.9%)	135(35.0%)	218(35.3%)
Heavy drinker	65(28.1%)	40(10.4%)	105(17.0%)
Total	231(37.5%)	386(62.5%)	617(100%)
Pearson Chi-sq	40	(p=0.0000)	

c- Drinking status in 1994 by age in 1994 (column %s)

Drinking status	Age 15 years	16 years	Total
Don't drink	153(36.6%)	69(34.7%)	222(36.0%)
Light drinker	173(41.4%)	65(32.7%)	238(38.6%)
Moderate drinker	70 16.7%)	52(26.1%)	122(19.8%)
Heavy drinker	22(5.3%)	13(6.5%)	35(5.7%)
Total	418(67.7%)	199(32.3%)	617(100%)
Pearson Chi-sq	9.19	(p=0.027)	

d- Drinking status in 1996 by age in 1996 (column %s)

Drinking status	Age 17 years	Age 18 years	Total
Don't drink	103(22.9%)	30(18.0%)	133(18.0%)
Light drinker	120(26.7%)	41(24.6%)	161(24.6%)
Moderate drinker	152(33.8%)	66(39.5%)	218(39.5%)
Heavy drinker	75(16.7%)	30(18.0%)	105(18.0%)
Total	450(72.9%)	167(27.1%)	617(100%)
Pearson Chi-sq	2.84	(p=0.42)	

e- Drink status in 1994 by Drinking status in 1996 (row %s)

Drinking status in 1994	Don't drink	up to 7 units	8-20 units	21+ units	Total
Don't drink	93(41.9%)	59(26.6%)	49(22.0%)	21(9.5%)	222(36.0%)
Light drinker	24(10.0%)	72(30.3%)	103(43.3%)	39(16.4%)	238(38.6%)
Moderate drinker	11(9.0%)	24(19.7%)	52(42.6%)	35(28.7%)	122(19.8%)
Heavy drinker	5(14.3%)	6(17.1%)	14(40%)	10(28.6%)	35(5.7%)
Total	133(21.6%)	161(26.1%)	218(35.3%)	105(17%)	617(100%)
Pearson Chi-sq	108	(p=0.0000)			

This data set provides only two time observations on a young adult's health-related behaviour. More linked observations on the individuals prior to 1994 and post-1996 are essential to enable us to unravel some of the complexities of interactions between life processes and whatever impact they may have on drinking status over time. However, even with two time observations per individual, we can illustrate how the application of appropriate statistical modelling of longitudinal observational data can provide added value from a statistical modelling perspective.

5.3.1.3. Statistical Analysis Using SABRE

The outcome variable is a categorical variable defining non-drinkers (1: those who reported consuming 0 units of alcohol), light drinkers (2: those who reported consuming between 1-8 units of alcohol), moderate drinkers (3: those who reported consuming between 9-20 units of alcohol), and heavy drinkers (4: those who reported consuming 21 units of alcohol or more). With a multi-category response variable and many independent variables, the common statistical approach is to fit a multinomial logistic regression model to the data. Further descriptive analyses of these data, in the form of cross-tabulations, provide evidence of high multicollinearity. For example, consider the variable 'worry' about money'. As shown in Tables 5.8(a-c), this variable is correlated with other variables such as 'happy with weight', 'best friend smokes' and 'at ease with opposite sex' as indicated by high chi-squared test statistic and corresponding small p-values. By now the reader should recognise that standard models such as the binary logistic regression are inappropriate for the analysis of longitudinal data. Furthermore, in comparison with the binary outcome of the teenage smoking example, the response variable for teenage drinking has four possible categories as stated above. The binary logistic model used in the teenage smoking example is a special case of the family of multinomial logistic models when the number of possible outcomes is two. The number of categories for the teenage drinking status variable is four. We cannot apply the binary logistic model directly, but we can apply an extended logistic model to these data, (see Chapter 2 and Appendix III). Once again, SABRE can fit such models. With us having only two time point, it is not practical for us to control for past behaviour in this case, though it is possible to do so in SABRE. A sample of the SABRE command file used to produce Tables 5.9 and 5.10 is provided in Sub-section 4.5.2. The interested reader is also referred to Appendix X for a complete list of SABRE commands.

Table 5.8(a-c). Example of multi-collinearity: Cross-classification of selected explanatory variables from the 1994 wave: frequencies (column percentages)

a.	Happy with weight		Total
Worry about money	put on/lose	happy	
Never	149 (44.3%)	151 (53.4%)	300 (49%)
A little	109 (32.4%)	91 (32.2%)	200 (32%)
A lot	78 (23.2%)	41 (14.5%)	119 (19%)
Total	336 (100%)	283 (100%)	619 (100%)
Pearson Chi-sq	8.66	(p=0.013)	

b.	Best friend smokes		Total
Worry about money	yes	no	
Never	125 (42.1%)	175 (54.3%)	300 (49%)
A little	102 (34.3%)	98 (30.4%)	200 (32%)
A lot	70 (23.6%)	49 (15.2%)	119 (19%)
Total	297 (100%)	322 (100%)	619 (100%)
Pearson Chi-sq	11.13	(p=0.004)	

c.	At ease with opposite sex		Total
Worry about money	yes	no	
Never	240 (47.3%)	60 (53.6%)	300 (49%)
A little	177 (34.9%)	23 (20.6%)	200 (32%)
A lot	90 (17.8%)	29 (25.9%)	119 (19%)
Total	507 (100%)	112 (100%)	619 (100%)
Pearson Chi-sq	9.77	(p=0.008)	

5.3.1.4. Interpretation of Results

A 'forward substitution' model-fitting procedure was adopted with the 'best' additional variable added to the model at each stage. The improvement in the model, as a result of adding each variable in turn, was assessed by a likelihood ratio test statistic denoted by the change in deviance. This process is shown in Table 5.9. To begin with, each variable is tested in the model on its own and its effect is noted. These effects are shown in the column headed 'null model'. In stage 1, age is chosen to enter the model over the variable 'used cannabis leaf'. The reason for this decision was to control for the effects of the better understood objective variable age before adding the other explanatory variables, as can be observed from the column headed 'model 1'. The consequence of adding age leads to a further nine variables ceasing to be statistically significant in stage 2. Note that both variables (age and 'used cannabis leaf') remain statistically significant and stay in the final model. The process was repeated in subsequent stages and the variable with the largest change in deviance was selected to enter the model until there were no remaining variables significant at the 5% significance level to add to the model. The parameter estimates for the first model are shown in Table 5.10. This table provides the list of selected explanatory variables and their categories, their parameter estimates and standard errors, chi-squared (χ^2) goodness of fit tests and their associated p-values. Positive estimates indicate likelihood of belonging to the non-drinker or light drinker categories, e.g. females are more likely to report lower units of alcohol consumption than males. Similarly, negative estimates indicate likelihood of belonging to moderate or heavy drinker categories, e.g. likelihood of heavy drinking increases with age.

The results, based on our sample, can be interpreted as follows:

- There are only nine explanatory variables in total that remained statistically significant.
- The likelihood of heavy drinking of alcohol appears to increase with age and parental involvement, whilst low consumption of alcohol appears to be related to: *not* experimenting with drugs including tobacco, ecstasy, amphetamines and cannabis; being a female; being a non-smoker; and being health conscious as measured by the variable 'considers health when choosing what to eat'.
- The most important aspect of these results is the statistically significant 'omitted variables' effect (ω) which suggests that there is substantial variation in drinking habits that is left unexplained by the observed explanatory variables.
-

5.3.1.5. Discussion

Over and above the observed measurements (selected explanatory variables in the model), the results from the above analysis suggest a highly statistically significant omitted variables effect (ω). Recall that ω is the standard deviation of the mixing distribution of the time-constant individual-specific random effect. A statistically significant ω suggests that substantial variation in the data has been left unexplained by the observed explanatory variables. Drinking habits may be subject to influence from unobserved environmental and socio-economic policies, and social/cultural pressures. For example, commonly, drinking initiations and exposure to alcohol drinking occur at home through parental and family lifestyle. Apart from family lifestyle, tobacco and alcohol, despite their negative economic, social and health consequences, are also well-established economic avenues for generating revenue by governments e.g. see [144-146]. The individual's *'freedom'* of choice has been a popular political justification for keeping this avenue open to the Treasury. However, since the 1970s, most governments caved in under pressure from scientists, health professionals and anti-smoking groups, and cigarette packets began to carry a health warning. Over subsequent decades, this health warning has developed into anti-smoking legislation to include, in some countries, a total ban on tobacco advertising, on the dispensing of tobacco products (vending machines), and on smoking in enclosed public places such as offices, cafes, restaurants and pubs. The extent of warnings about the consumption of alcohol appears to have followed a reverse pattern: not only are there no health warnings visible on alcoholic drink containers but

Table 5.9. Teenage drinking patterns: variable selection process

Explanatory Variables	d.f	Null model Deviance	Model 1 Deviance	Model 2 Deviance	Model 3 Deviance	Model 4 Deviance	Model 5 Deviance	Model 6 Deviance	Final Model Deviance
Sex	1	13.54	14.00	21.6	31.58	30	31.64	IN	30.92
Age	4	133.64	IN	IN	IN	IN	IN	IN	14.36
How fit are you?	2	2.98	out	-	-	-	-	-	-
If you drink at home do your parents know?	3	129.18	111.48	IN	IN	IN	IN	IN	116.02
Do you smoke?	1	126.88	93.52	87.88	IN	IN	IN	IN	34.08
At least one in family smokes	1	8.4	8.42	8.6	2.1	-	-	-	-
Best friend smokes	2	110.74	80.00	85.4	46.2	32.24	IN	IN	29.98
Main source of information	4	38.46	16.76	17.74	11.26	7.26	-	-	-
Worry about school?	2	2.88	out	-	-	-	-	-	-
Worry about money matters?	2	49.62	12.42	10.76	4.24	-	-	-	-
Worry about health?	2	0.22	out	-	-	-	-	-	-
Worry about career?	2	1.8	out	-	-	-	-	-	-
Worry about unemployment?	2	2.16	out	-	-	-	-	-	-
Worry about friends?	2	0.12	out	-	-	-	-	-	-
Worry about family?	2	2.42	out	-	-	-	-	-	-
Worry about your look?	2	0.1	out	-	-	-	-	-	-
Worry about drugs?	2	8.02	7.32	6.08	1.04	-	-	-	-
Worry about AIDs?	2	14.08	16.12	12.16	7.34	7.22	3.8	-	-
In charge of own health?	2	2.64	out	-	-	-	-	-	-
Health is just luck?	2	5.12	1.94	-	-	-	-	-	-
Take care of own health?	2	5.68	1.72	-	-	-	-	-	-
Easily get ill?	2	13.06	6.00	5.88	-	-	-	-	-

Explanatory Variables	d.f	Null model Deviance	1 Deviance	2 Deviance	3 Deviance	4 Deviance	5 Deviance	6 Deviance	Final Model Deviance
Have you used amphetamines?	1	130.32	55.32	52.84	32.82	12.5	8.6	IN	4.22
Have you used barbiturates?	1	8.44	2.70	out	-	-	-	-	-
Have you used cannabis resin?	1	134.92	70.96	67.94	30.82	8.78	7.74	2.36	-
Have you used cannabis leaf?	1	180.98	86.18	83	46.94	IN	IN	IN	12.44
Have you used ecstasy?	1	114.76	40.92	41.86	25.54	10.54	8.84	4.72	5.7
Have you used coke?	1	12.12	1.78	out	-	-	-	-	-
Have you used crack?	1	5.66	0.76	out	-	-	-	-	-
Have you used natural hallucigent?	1	68.68	34.30	31.42	15.6	4.78	-	-	-
Have you used synthetic hallucigent?	1	100.82	58.62	53.70	28.48	12.48	10	4.78	-
Have you used heroin?	1	19.4	7.14	8.78	5.72	3.74	-	-	-
Have you used solvents?	1	41.86	20.08	19.50	7.88	2.4	-	-	-
Have you used tranquilisers?	1	8.82	1.96	out	-	-	-	-	-
Do you have breakfast?	1	10.00	3.24	out	-	-	-	-	-
Consider health when choosing food?	2	10.46	12.92	13.82	14	11.46	12.68	10.44	11.42
Happy with your weight?	2	7.08	4.96	out	-	-	-	-	-

Table 5.10. Teenage drinking pattern: model fitting results

Explanatory Variables	Parameter estimates	Standard Error	Significance level
Sex			<<0.0005
Male	0.00		
Female	0.76	0.14	
Age			0.001
14	0.00		
15	-0.29	0.18	
16	-0.66	0.15	
17	-0.74	0.20	
If you drink at home do your parents know?			<<0.00005
Do not drink alcohol	0.00		
Parents always/usually know	-2.18	0.22	
Parents sometimes/never know	-1.91	0.27	
Missing	-1.56	0.47	
Is a smoker			<<0.0005
No	0.00		
Yes	-0.88	0.16	
Best friend is a smoker			<0.0005
No	0.00		
Yes	-0.73	0.14	
Drug experiments: Amphetamines			0.05
No	0.00		
Yes	-0.42	0.20	
Drug experiments: cannabis leaf			0.001
No	0.00		
Yes	-0.56	0.16	
Drug experiments: ecstasy			0.05
No	0.00		
Yes	0.50	0.21	
Do you consider health when choosing what you eat?			0.005
Never	0.00		
Sometimes	0.60	0.22	
Quite often/Always	0.27	0.22	
Scale parameter (ω)	0.72	0.15	

also drinking appears to be encouraged through all media, in particular the entertainment medium [171]. In most western societies, alcoholic beverages may be consumed anywhere and anytime. Furthermore, the 'happy hour', when alcohol may be purchased at half price, is a regular feature in most clubs and pubs. Governments, health ministries and health promotion schemes appear to recommend guidelines for *safe* alcohol consumption. Commonly, most anti-drinking campaigns are often associated with drink-driving prevention schemes. In New Zealand, the message of the anti-drinking campaign explicitly declares 'it is not the drinking, it is how we drink'. Additional encouragement appears to come from an unlikely source: the medical profession's proclamation that alcohol is a preventive agent against heart disease through the popular media.

Notwithstanding the social culture of drinking as discussed above, in behavioural studies, the possibility of a past behaviour effect (e.g. state dependence and duration dependence) should not be discounted. It would have been preferable to follow up pupils from an earlier age before the onset of drinking, and to collect observations on more than two time points, thereby allowing us to incorporate past behaviour, pathways to drinking, and other dynamics of behaviour into the analysis. Furthermore, the individual-specific error term accounting for heterogeneity is time-constant. Thus, the model does not account for time-varying heterogeneity (such as the feel good factor). Some of these limitations, such as not accounting for time-varying heterogeneity, may be overcome by adopting a pragmatic multi-method approach, e.g. see [29, 63].

However, the purpose of this chapter is to demonstrate the effects of omitted variables on the estimates of parameters in standard logistic and logistic-normal random effects models. As noted in Chapter 1, when using survey-type data to investigate the relationship between smoking and explanatory variables, a number of analytical issues must be addressed. Also noted in Sub-section 5.3.1 was the large number of factors that have been associated with teenage drinking. How the explanatory variables are associated with each other (e.g. see Tables 5.7a-c) will have an impact on the final results. Multicollinearity can be addressed within the statistical modelling framework we have adopted. One of the major difficulties with survey-type studies is how to take into account residual heterogeneity (inherent variation due to omitted variables).

Survey studies often treat a range of factors (e.g. parental smoking/drinking behaviour and self-esteem, psychological and environmental measures) as independent correlates of drinking (i.e. that no other effects are present). Such an approach ignores the consequences of both multicollinearity and residual heterogeneity.

One of the main challenges facing researchers, practitioners and policy makers must surely be how to inform the process of decision/policy-making. Health promotion programmes must be based on reliable evidence from appropriate longitudinal research designs. Complexities arise usually as a result of ignoring substantive issues (e.g subjectivity, objectivity and residual heterogeneity) leading to mis-specification, mis-interpretation and misleading conclusions. Preventional policies that are based on cross-sectional surveys, or which focus on certain variables such as peer pressure, often fail to take into account the complex dynamic behaviour of the young individuals themselves. Such policies often focus on influencing the 'action' indicated by a variable rather than the underlying effect that the variable represents. Furthermore, an evaluation programme is very rarely integrated within interventional and preventional health promotion policies.

5.3.1.6. Summary

With survey or observational studies, it is possible to measure a wide range of individual, social and environmental variables. It is inevitable that within the same survey, there will be objective variables as well as subjectively measured variables. On the other hand, some other variables, such as personality and social attrition, are unobserved leading to complex inter-relationships and interactions in data requiring additional complexities in the methodology. In studying dynamic social behaviour such as drinking and smoking, it is essential to adopt appropriate study design, data and analytical methodologies. An appropriate study design would incorporate substantive issues related to the dynamics of the process under investigation. For example, standard statistical methods such as logistic regression may be applied effectively to cross-sectional data, but cannot be utilised to exploit fully the richness of longitudinal data. In this example, we have demonstrated that, through the appropriate application of statistical modelling, as in most social processes, there will be substantial residual heterogeneity in the data due to omitted variables. Therefore, caution must be exercised when interpreting results. In the context of drinking, however, the underlying drinking culture, that is intertwined with other processes (e.g. economic policies, the entertainment industry, social attitudes to drinking alcohol), provides the explanatory power of the model. Study design, analysis and interpretation of results and health/social policy formation must take into account the culture of drinking alcohol.

5.4. EXAMPLE 3: BIVARIATE BINARY RESPONSE

5.4.1. Linguistic Innovation in London

5.4.1.1. Background

The authors of this study [31] considered whether ethnicity is a significant determinant of variation in the spoken English of young working class people in London. The analysis is based on a corpus of 1.4 million words of transcribed interviews with 100 people aged 16-19 and 16 elderly speakers in their 70s and 80s from one inner London borough and from one outer London borough. Many (mainly white) Londoners moved from the inner city (the 'East End') to outer London and further afield, particularly Essex, in the 1950s; by contrast, the inner London borough has a high proportion of recent immigrants from overseas. The study explores whether the nature of a speaker's friendship group is a key factor in the diffusion of linguistic innovations, and whether this factor interacts with ethnicity. Thus the study hypothesizes that speakers draw on a range of linguistic forms that cannot necessarily, or at least can no longer, be attributed to specific ethnic groups. In other words, the wider or more diverse the network of friends, the less distinct will be the accent of the speaker, the harder it will be for the listener to identify ethnicity and location of the speaker.

5.4.1.2. Data

The data for this study came from the project *Linguistic innovators: the English of adolescents in London* (see [31]), with informants from two boroughs: Hackney (inner London) and Havering (outer London). The localities were selected on the basis of demographic and social differences: Hackney is ethnically very diverse and economically relatively deprived, while Havering is an area with higher mobility and higher levels of prosperity.

In this study design, the speech of a group of speakers (see Table 5.11) was recorded and played back to a sample of listeners. After listening, the listeners were required to make a guess on the ethnicity of the speaker (White, Black, Asian or Other) and the locality (Hackney or Havering) they came from. The outcomes comprised two possible sets of binary observations: (i) the listeners guessed ethnicity correctly (yes=1) or did not guess correctly (no=0); (ii) the listeners guessed locality correctly (yes=1) or did not guess correctly (no=0). This type of data, which comprises two parallel binary response variables, is called bivariate binary response data. SABRE may be used to fit a bivariate binary logit model to such data (see Sub-section 4.5.3).

Table 5.11. Background characteristics of the speakers

Speaker	Sex	Locality	Ethnicity	Friendship network score
Megan	Female	Hackney	Anglo ('White')	3 (mainly Anglo network)
Andrew	Male	Hackney	Anglo ('White')	3 (mainly Anglo network)
Laura	Female	Hackney	Anglo ('White')	5 (multiethnic network)

Table 5.11.- (Continued)

Ryan	Male	Hackney	Anglo ('White')	5 (multiethnic network)
Sulema	Female	Hackney	Non-Anglo ('Other')	5 (multiethnic network)
Kirsty	Female	Hackney	Non-Anglo ('Asian')	5 (multiethnic network)
Grace	Female	Hackney	Non-Anglo ('Black')	5 (multiethnic network)
Dom	Male	Hackney	Non-Anglo ('Other')	4 (multiethnic network)
Amjad	Male	Hackney	Non-Anglo ('Asian')	5 (multiethnic network)
Chris	Male	Hackney	Non-Anglo ('Black')	5 (multiethnic network)
Kelly	Female	Havering	Anglo ('White')	2 (mainly Anglo network)
Dale	Male	Havering	Anglo ('White')	2 (mainly Anglo network)

In addition, the study collected data on the speaker's ethnicity and their network of friends. Although the main theme of the study was the hypothesis that the linguistic features are influenced by the diversity of network, the same could be argued about the listeners. In other words, the ability to guess correctly the ethnicity and locality of a speaker is conditional upon the level of exposure to a diversity of accents. This dataset does not lend itself to controlling for listener's characteristics. Nevertheless we may proceed with the analysis using SABRE.

5.4.1.3. Statistical Analysis Using SABRE

There are two parallel responses with two possible outcomes each, namely ethnicity correctly identified (1) or not (0), and locality correctly identified (1) or not (0). Clearly, the application of a standard logistic model to parallel outcomes is inappropriate. A pragmatic approach would be to fit separate logistic models to each binary response and to compare and triangulate the results from the various models. However, SABRE may be used to fit a single model, a bivariate binary model to such data (see Sub-section 4.5.3). Due to the small number of explanatory variables, the variable selection process started by fitting the full model i.e. the model which included all the explanatory variables. The model fitting results are shown in Table 5.12.

5.4.1.4. Interpretation of Results

Several models were fitted to the data. Here we report the results of fitting three models. The reader is referred to Cheshire et al. [31] for full details of the analysis. In the analysis reported in this section, stimulus_number has been declared as the random effect which will allow for residual heterogeneity; that is, the inherent variation between stimuli, or speakers.

The first model is the standard logit model with the assumption that the two binary responses are independent of each other. The results for this model are shown under the heading 'Standard; Uncorrelated' of Table 5.12. The second model also assumes independence in the bivariate responses but incorporates a random effect. The results for this model are shown under the heading 'With random effect; Uncorrelated' of Table 5.12. The third model is also a random effects model but drops the independence assumption and assumes that the bivariate responses are correlated. The results for this model are shown under the heading 'With random effect; Correlated' of Table 5.12.

The first striking feature of table 5.12 is that the standard model appears to overestimate the significance of the explanatory variables. Their parameter estimates are robust from one model to another, but their corresponding standard errors are smaller in the standard model than in the random effects models.

Table 5.12. Model fitting results for bivariate binary response data

	Standard		With random effect			
	Uncorrelated		Uncorrelated		Correlated	
Explanatory Variables	p.e	s.e	p.e	s.e	p.e	s.e
r1 (ethnicity)	0.46	0.417	0.44	1.117	0.42	1.119
Sex	0.92	0.221	0.98	0.623	0.98	0.624
Network3	-0.66	0.433	-0.74	1.174	-0.75	1.176
Network4	-2.67	0.503	-2.73	1.312	-2.73	1.315
Network5	-2.36	0.400	-2.43	1.055	-2.42	1.057
r2 (location)	-0.37	0.390	-0.34	0.522	-0.35	0.529
Sex	-0.39	0.245	-0.42	0.317	-0.41	0.322
Network3	1.75	0.394	1.78	0.532	1.77	0.540
Network4	2.47	0.510	2.50	0.649	2.50	0.657
Network5	2.38	0.372	2.46	0.500	2.46	0.507
Scale1			0.85	0.216	0.86	0.217
Scale2			0.28	0.164	0.29	0.167
Correlation					0.19	0.489

The second feature is that the scale parameters `scale1` and `scale2` both appear to be significant in both random effects models, this indicates that indicating a significant amount of variation in both binary responses between stimuli (speakers) has been left unexplained by those explanatory variables included in the model. The correlation parameter is not significant, indicating that the odds of a listener correctly identifying the ethnicity of a stimulus (speaker) are not significantly associated with the chances of that listener succeeding in getting the location correct.

The sex effect does not appear to be statistically significant and the effect of network is considerably reduced in the two random effects models. The third feature is that network appears to be statistically significant. The results for network suggest that it is easier to **identify correctly a speaker's ethnicity** if the friendship network score is low, but more difficult to identify correctly where a speaker comes from.

5.4.1.5. Summary

To **address the issue of listeners' background characteristics and exposure** to a diversity of accents, the listener ID variable was declared as the random effect in place of stimulus_number (results not shown here). The third model, when the independence assumption is dropped, reported a perfect negative correlation (-1) for the bivariate binary responses. If the listener guessed one of the responses right, s/he would get the other one wrong. In other words, if the listeners guessed ethnicity right then they guessed the location wrong. This may be indicative of a number of social and behavioural issues, e.g. stereotyping. For example, an accent that is associated with the more deprived locations or with the non-white population may influence the listener to guess the lower socio-economic locality as the choice for location.

An interesting feature of Table 5.12 is that network appears to be negatively associated with ethnicity but positively related to location. This indicates that the nature/type of locality may influence or be the reason for the diversity of networking and friends. An area which, to all intents and purposes, could be defined as homogeneous is less likely to provide opportunities for networking and friendship across different ethnic groups than another area which is heterogeneous and more cosmopolitan.

Clearly, further research is needed to investigate the dynamics of changes and shifts in linguistic innovation given the shift in societies not only from a mono-culture to a multi-cultural society but also from a language-based culture to a more technology-based culture [180] with the advent of emails, mobile phones and text messaging.

Chapter 6

CONCLUSIONS

In this book, we have demonstrated that the dynamics of a process cannot be interpreted in terms of simple transitional probabilities from one state to another, e.g. from low morale at time one to high morale in the next time point. We have demonstrated the necessity for statistical control in the analysis. In addition, we have also demonstrated the need for critical selection of the method for analysis. For instance, recall the analysis of survival in old age (Chapter 2). In the first analysis, where survival was a binary outcome, the appropriate statistical technique was applied to the data. However, as explained in Chapter 2, there may be within-group dissimilarities, i.e. those who died at the start of the study period may be very different to those who died 4 or 8 years later. The application of a logit model is appropriate but the binary grouping only distinguishes between survivors and the deceased, i.e. those who were alive at the time of repeat interview and those who had died. This issue was then addressed by refining the data and consequently by adding complexity to the method of analysis, i.e. by applying the multinomial response model and carrying out time series analysis. In the multinomial model, a distinction was made within the survivor group to create a third group, i.e. those who were alive but in residential care. In the time series analysis, dates of death were used to calculate survival times. We were then able to model the durations survived by the individuals. The point that arises is that we were able to refine the modelling because of the availability of data. In most cases, data do not lend themselves to the application of complex models which are required in order to address issues of dynamics. In other words, we may be unable to continue modelling beyond the standard logistic model without additional data. We can, however, use our knowledge of the substantive issues to: (i) exercise caution when interpreting the results; (ii) be pragmatic and explore the data to ascertain the existence of complex interactions between observed variables and between observed and unobserved variables.

To illustrate this point further, consider the teenage smoking example. Prior to phase two data on teenage smoking becoming available, cross-sectional data from phase one were already available and an analysis of these data had been reported to the relevant authority. Here we reproduce this analysis in Tables 6.1 and 6.2.

As discussed in Chapter 5, the smoking variable is a binary response (smoker/non-smoker). Therefore, it was appropriate to apply a standard binary logistic model to the data. The model building process led to the variables listed in Table 6.1 being selected for inclusion in the model. First, the 24 variables that were tested individually at the start of the modelling process were all highly significant. After allowing control for other variables, half of the variables ceased to be significant (see [29] for full details of the analysis). Second, Table 6.1, although correct, does not tell the whole story. It is quite easy to conclude from Table 6.1 that 'best friend' has the largest effect on smoking followed by the variables 'have partner', 'how feel with opposite sex', 'which parent live with', and the two 'worrying' variables. The results in Table 6.1 also suggest that, compared to their respective reference groups, the odds of being a smoker increased for those who claimed their best friend smoked (odds ratio 14.58, 95% confidence interval 12.63-16.83), to have a partner (odds ratio 3.41, 95% confidence interval 2.36-4.92), to be at ease with the opposite sex (odds ratio 1.80, 95% confidence interval 1.37 to 2.36), to worry a lot about money problems (odds ratio 1.71, 95% confidence interval 1.43-2.05) and to worry a lot about family problems (odds ratio 1.37, 95% confidence interval 1.15-162). On the other hand, the odds of being a smoker decreased for those who claimed to be happy with their body shape (odds ratio 0.75, 95% confidence interval 0.65-0.87) and those who claimed to consider their health often when choosing food (odds ratio 0.50, 95% confidence interval 0.39-0.63). Pupils who lived with foster parents appeared to have an increased risk of nearly four times that of pupils who lived with both parents. The result for 'which parent live with' can be explained as past behaviour leading to a selection bias; it is plausible that smoking may well have started while in care prior to placement with foster parents [181].

An understanding of the dynamics of human behaviour motivated further exploration of the results. It is surprising that a pragmatic approach could be used to gain further insight into the process. In other words, the role that different variables play in determining smoking behaviour can be examined by comparing results from the three models in Table 6.2. The inclusion of socio-environmental factors (model 2) has a major impact on the significance of the demographic variables that were included in model 1 (Table 6.2). There are marked changes in the parameter estimates of the variables 'gender', 'age' and 'which parent live with'. The variables reflecting social status, 'where live' and 'social class', are no longer significant and drop out of the model. While some increases in parameter estimates are to be expected when adding new significant variables to the logistic regression model, the large decrease in parameter estimates confirms that the effects of the variables 'age' and 'which parent live with' have been reduced substantially. This is consistent with the socio-environmental variables having an intervening effect between age, parent(s) and smoking. Similarly, when the socio-psychological variables are added to model 2 (model 3, Table 6.2), a modest decrease in the parameter estimates of the demographic and socio-environmental variables can be noted. This decrease is consistent with the socio-psychological factors having an intervening effect between the demographic and socio-environmental variables and smoking.

The variables 'self-esteem', 'worrying about school' and 'whether happy with weight', which were significant on their own, failed to remain in the final model after controlling for other variables. On the other hand, the variable 'being happy with body shape' remained significant and was included in the final model. It is therefore plausible that the variable 'being happy with body shape' may reflect the respondents' state of mind at the time of the interview, regardless of actual body shape and weight. This means that, in addition to body shape, the variable 'happy with body shape' may well be an indication of this group's insensitivity to social pressures; that is, the social influences that may lead to smoking (e.g.

see also [155]). In particular, individuals with a similar body shape may have different outcomes: some become smokers and some do not.

It can be seen that the change in the parameter estimate of the variable 'best friend smokes' from model 2 to model 3 (Table 6.2) is over two times its standard error. This change is consistent with the variable 'best friend' having an intervening effect between smoking and the demographic variables. If there is a 'true' best friend effect, it is too complex to identify with cross-sectional data. As discussed in Section 5.2, it is plausible that, prior to taking up smoking, such pupils may have had a lower self-esteem, a wish to gain confidence, a desire to belong to a peer group and possibly lacked social and parental guidance. There is some evidence to suggest that parental influence indirectly predicts lower levels of smoking [151-153]. The 'best friend' effect may not be straightforward to interpret with these data because we have no knowledge of these pupils' previous smoking habits; a pupil may have been a smoker prior to the friendship. Furthermore, the high odds ratio for 'best friend' may well be inflated due to a pragmatic sampling strategy. Surveying of all pupils within classrooms in selected schools may have achieved a maximum response, but has added complexities to the data, e.g. (i) the clustering effect where pupils with similar outcome characteristics tend to form clusters (or social groups), and (ii) the possibility of double counting where pupils in the same classroom cite each other as their best friend (e.g. see [182]). Cross-sectional analysis of such data will lead to an artificially inflated effect of 'best friend' on smoking (e.g. see [14]). Therefore, it is unwise to interpret 'best friend' directly as a peer pressure effect.

The result for the variable 'how feels with opposite sex' in Table 6.1 suggests that feeling at ease with the opposite sex increases the likelihood of being a smoker which may imply that 'more confident' pupils are likely to smoke. On the other hand, Table 6.2 suggests the possibility of a more dynamic social process (notice the changes in the parameter estimates of variables in model 3 compared with those in model 2). Once again, we have no knowledge either of the pupils' past smoking behaviour or of past patterns of their social interactions with the opposite sex. Therefore, it would be unwise to interpret the result for this variable as any causal relationship between confidence and smoking.

From the results in Tables 6.1 and 6.2, similar conclusions can be made for the variables 'considers health when choosing food', 'worry about money problems' and 'worry about family problems'. These three variables were statistically significant and remained in the final model. As most pupils have been made aware of the dangers of smoking, these variables may be a proxy for the underlying effect of attitudes to health and smoking. The choice of food represents the health consciousness of pupils, suggesting that those who attach importance to health-related behaviour have a reduced risk of being a smoker, while the 'worry' variables serve to demonstrate the subjective effect of smoking, where smoking leads to the maintenance of smoking [132, 138]. Again, without prior information on the pupils' smoking behaviour, these results do not constitute evidence that worrying leads to smoking. This association between smoking and worrying/health may help to explain the prevalence, but not incidence, of smoking.

It appears that those pupils who have or have had a partner (boyfriend or girlfriend) are more likely to be a smoker than those who have never had a partner. It is not clear whether having a partner is the reason for pupils' smoking habits, or whether young people smoke to be sociable. However, from the results shown in Table 6.2, while there is a small change in the parameter estimates of the objective variables from model 2 to model 3, the change in the parameter estimates of the socio-environmental variables is around twice their standard error. It is therefore plausible that the variable 'have a partner' may be reflecting a 'best friend' effect or a 'foster parent' effect, as discussed earlier.

Table 6.1. Standard logistic regression: odds ratios of smoking with their respective 95% confidence limits after controlling for other factors

Explanatory variables	Lower	Odds Ratio	Upper
Age (baseline: 12-13)			
14-15	1.59	1.84	2.13
Sex (baseline: Male)			
Female	1.68	1.96	2.30
Which parent live with			
Both parents	1.00	1.00	1.00
Mother only	0.92	1.13	1.40
Father only	0.92	1.45	2.31
Mother and step-father	1.18	1.48	1.84
Father and step-mother	0.78	1.31	2.19
Foster parents	1.78	3.74	7.87
Other	0.79	1.31	2.14
Whether drinks			
No	1.00	1.00	1.00
Yes	2.19	2.56	3.00
Whether at least one family smokes			
No	1.00	1.00	1.00
Yes	1.40	1.62	1.89
Best friend smokes			
No	1.00	1.00	1.00
Yes	12.23	14.16	16.36
Have partner			
Never had one	1.00	1.00	1.00
Not at the moment	1.44	2.02	2.85
Yes, few weeks	2.25	3.25	4.71
Yes, up to 6 months	3.21	4.77	7.09
Yes, up to a year	1.72	2.80	4.53
Yes, more than 1 year	2.10	3.17	4.78
How feel with opposite sex			
Very uneasy	1.00	1.00	1.00
A little uneasy	1.01	1.32	1.74
At ease	1.43	1.89	2.49
Happy with body shape			
No	1.00	1.00	1.00
Yes	0.69	0.80	0.93
Considers health when choosing food			
Never	1.00	1.00	1.00
Sometimes	0.50	0.62	0.77
Quite often	0.38	0.48	0.62
Very often	0.23	0.32	0.43
Always	0.30	0.44	0.63
Worry about money problems			
Never/hardly ever	1.00	1.00	1.00
A little	1.12	1.33	1.58
Quite a lot/a lot	1.43	1.71	2.05
Worry about family problems			
Never/hardly ever	1.00	1.00	1.00
A little	0.97	1.17	1.42
Quite a lot/a lot	1.15	1.37	1.62

Table 6.2. Model fitting results for the smoking data - N=9230

	Model 1		Model 2		Model 3	
Explanatory variables	p.e.	s.e.	p.e.	s.e.	p.e.	s.e.
Demographic factors						
Age (baseline: 12-13)						
14-15	1.06	0.06	0.68	0.07	0.61	0.08
Sex (baseline: Male)						
Female	0.52	0.06	0.68	0.07	0.67	0.08
Which parent live with						
Both parents	0.00		0.00		0.00	
Mother only	0.47	0.08	0.23	0.10	0.12	0.11
Father only	0.69	0.18	0.49	0.23	0.37	0.24
Mother and step-father	0.80	0.09	0.53	0.11	0.39	0.11
Father and step-mother	0.77	0.20	0.44	0.25	0.27	0.26
Foster parents	1.63	0.29	1.56	0.37	1.32	0.38
Other	0.73	0.19	0.38	0.24	0.28	0.25
Where live						
Town/city centre	0.00					
Town/city suburb	-0.30	0.13				
Small town/city centre	-0.08	0.11				
Small town/Suburb	-0.26	0.11				
In village	0.10	0.10				
Outside town/village	0.20	0.13				
Social class						
High	0.00					
Medium	0.15	0.10				
Low	0.25	0.09				
Socio-environmental factors						
Whether drinks						
No			0.00		0.00	
Yes			1.11	0.08	0.94	0.08
Whether at least one family smokes						
No			0.00		0.00	
Yes			0.60	0.08	0.47	0.08
Best friend smokes						
No			0.00		0.00	
Yes			2.81	0.07	2.65	0.07
Socio-psychological factors						
Have partner						
Never had one					0.00	
Not at the moment					0.70	0.17
Yes, few weeks					1.18	0.19
Yes, up to 6 months					1.56	0.20
Yes, up to a year					1.03	0.25
Yes, more than 1 year					1.15	0.21
How feel with opposite sex						
Very uneasy					0.00	
A little uneasy					0.28	0.14
At ease					0.64	0.14
Happy with body shape						
No					0.00	
Yes					-0.22	0.08
Worry about money problems						
Never/hardly ever					0.00	
A little					0.29	0.09
Quite a lot/a lot					0.54	0.09
Worry about family problems						
Never/hardly ever					0.00	
A little					0.16	0.10
Quite a lot/a lot					0.31	0.09

In order to be able to have confidence in the results from studies of human behaviour, the issues relating to the dynamics of behaviour must be explored within the study framework. A common argument for excluding a discussion of such issues is to use the context of the study or a lack of access to longitudinal data. As demonstrated in this book, a discussion of such important issues serves to improve the study and to aid the interpretation of results. Whether we like it or not, regardless of the type of data or context, the issues concerning dynamics do exist. It is better to incorporate them into the study and analysis than to ignore them, even though the study itself may be cross-sectional. Appropriate methodologies must be adopted to cope with the complex issues which may arise throughout the study process, from design to data collection, analysis and interpretation. Even when we are limited to dealing with cross-sectional data and analysis, the issues concerning dynamics will not disappear!

The above issues can be explored by returning to the cross-sectional analysis of the teenage smoking data. **Recall the 'best friend' effect and the effects from other subjective variables.** We adopted a pragmatic approach by grouping the explanatory variables according to their types; namely demographic, socio-environmental and socio-psychological (see Table 6.2). A comparison of three different models based on the above grouping of explanatory variables enabled us to explore the effect of model mis-specification. This additional exploratory analysis **indicated that the 'best friend' effect may not be as strong as it appears in the literature. The 'best friend' effect may owe its significance to omitted variables, possible clustering** or a selection bias effect where similarity attracts, i.e. smokers are more likely to become friends with other smokers and similarly non-smokers are more likely to befriend non-smokers. More importantly, these preliminary findings were confirmed by the longitudinal modelling in Chapter 5.

As discussed in Chapter 1, the first issues to consider relate to the nature of the data under scrutiny and measurement definition. Whether it is clinical or social survey measurement, an important aspect is defining and measuring variables appropriately. For example, can we measure quality of life simply in terms of access to TV and video/DVD players, computers, games machines (e.g. **xbox) and number of cars? Comparisons of 'haves' and 'have-nots'** only produce relative material gain indicators that may not have much to do with quality of life. Another important issue to remember is that, in most studies, we are bound by what can be observed and measured. Often, we ignore the importance of those variables or factors that are unmeasurable, difficult to measure or simply omitted from the study, e.g. personality, the feel good factor and frailty. We cannot address the issue of omitted variables directly within a cross-sectional study but that does not mean that such important issues can be ignored or would not exist even if the study were cross-sectional, see Figure 1.7. In a formal multivariate analysis, omitted variables are often the source of model mis-specification.

In terms of informing the process of policy development, some variables are easy to interpret. For example, consider the 'district nurse' effect from the survival analysis in Chapter 2 and the 'foster parent' effect from the teenage smoking example in Chapter 5. Both indicate a negative association: those elderly in receipt of a district nurse service were more likely to die; youths living with foster parents were more likely to be smokers. An examination of the datasets revealed that these results are not unexpected and are related to selection bias and past behaviour rather than direct effects from district nurse or foster parents. Those elderly who received a district nurse care service were more likely to be dependent and frail than those who did not have this service, and the youths living with foster parents were more likely to have picked up their smoking habit prior to placement with foster parents. In other words, there is no evidence of cause and effect, i.e. receiving the district nurse care service does not cause death but may be an indicator of impending death. Other variables are not so easy to explain and reflect a more complex inter-relationship between the observed explanatory variables, omitted variables and outcome variables. Looking at Table 6, we may be inclined to interpret the results as: older female pupils who drink and whose best friend smokes, who are not happy with their body shape, who do not consider their health when choosing food, who worry about problems, who are living with one parent and who are exposed to family members who smoke, are more likely to be smokers. Taken at face value, such results are more confusing and are not likely to increase insight into the process of teenage smoking. For example, do we develop health promotion policies that increase pupils' income and that fence them off from exposure to smoking through their family and friends? And how do we help to make young people feel happy about their body shape? To effect change in perception and behaviour both at the individual level and across society, requires policy changes in all other social processes, e.g. politics, media, education, economy. Policy makers appear to pick out those variables that can be manipulated independently of other variables, e.g. in the past, the **emphasis has been on the effects from 'best friend' and parents** on smoking habits. Thus, policies that attempt to sever one social link with smoking may actually help to exaggerate the effects from other factors through the feedback effect and the other issues discussed in this book.

REFERENCES

[1] Short S. Elective Affinities: Research and Health Policy Development. In: Gardner H, ed. *Health Policy in Australia*. Melbourne: Oxford University Press; 1997.
[2] Wenger GC. *The Supportive Network - coping with old age*. London: George Allen and Unwin; 1984.
[3] Beautrais AL. *Serious suicide attempts in young people: a case control study* [PhD]. Christchurch: Dept. of Psycholigical Medicine, Christchurch School of Medicine; 1996.
[4] Beautrais AL. Suicides and serious suicide attempts: two populations or one? *Psychol. Med.* 2001;31:837-45.
[5] Beautrais AL, Joyce PR, Mulder RT. The Canterbury suicide project: Aims, overview and progress. *Community Mental Health in New Zealand.* 1994;8(2):32-39.
[6] Khan A, Warner HA, Brown WA. Symptom Reduction and Suicide Risk in Patients Treated With Placebo in Antidepressant Clinical Trials: An Analysis of the Food and Drug Administration Database. *Arch. Gen. Psychiatry.* 2000;57:311-17.
[7] Hall WD, Mant A, Mitchell PB, Rendle VA, Hickie IB, McManus P. Association between antidepressant prescribing and suicide in Australia, 1991-2000: trend analysis. *BMJ.* 2003;326.
[8] Shahtahmasebi S. Suicides by Mentally Ill People. *TheScientificWorldJOURNAL.* 2003;3:684-93.
[9] Shahtahmasebi S. Suicide in New Zealand. In: Merrick J, Zalsman G, eds. *Suicidal behavior in adolescence. An international perspective*. New York: Freund Publishing; 2005.
[10] Chamberlain G. Panel Data. *Handbook of Economics.* Vol. 21984:Chapter 22.
[11] Heckman J. Statistical models for discrete panel data. In: Manski C, McFadden D, eds. *Structural Analysis of Discrete Data with Econometric Applications*. Cambridge, Mass: MIT press; 1981.
[12] Davies R, Martin AM, Penn R. Linear modelling with clustered observations an illustratative example of earnings in the engineering industry. *Environment and Planning A.* 1988;20:1069-84.
[13] Davies RB, Pickles AR. Robustness in modelling dynamics of choice. In: Hauer J, Timmermans H, Wrigley N, eds. *Contemporary Developments in Quantitative Geography*. Dordrecht, the Netherlands: D Reidel; 1987.
[14] Davies RB. The limitation of cross-sectional analysis. In: Crouchley R, ed. *Longitudinal Data Analysis*. London: Sage; 1987.

[15] Pickles AR, Davies RB. Inference from cross-sectional and longitudinal data for dynamic behavioural processes. In: Hauer J, ed. *Urban dynamics and spatial choice behaviour*: Kluwer Academic; 1989:81-104.

[16] Davies RB, Pickles AR. Longitudinal versus cross-sectional methods for behavioural research: a first-round knockout. *Environment and Planning A*. 1985;17:1315-29.

[17] Berridge D, Santos DM. Modelling ordinal recurrent events. *Survey and Statistical Modelling*. 1996:233-40.

[18] Lancaster T, Nickell S. The analysis of re-employment probabilities for the unemployed. *Journal of the Royal Statistical Association*. 1980;Series A; 14(3):141-65.

[19] Wallace D, Silver JL. *Econometrics - An introduction*. New York: Addison-Wesley; 1988.

[20] Wenger GC. Morale in old age: A review of the literature. *Int. J. Geriatr. Psychiat.* 1992;7:699-708.

[21] Adams RG. Emotional closeness and physical distance between friends: implications for elderly women living in age-segregated and age-integrated settings. *International J. Aging and Human Development*. 1985;221.

[22] Massy WF, Montgomery DB, Morrison DG. *Stochastic Models of Buying Behaviour*: The MIT Press; 1970.

[23] McCullagh P, Nelder JA. *Generalised Linear Models*. London: Chapman and Hall; 1983.

[24] Aitkin M, Anderson D, Francis B, Hinde J. *Statistical modelling in GLIM*. Oxford: Oxford University Press; 1989.

[25] Davies RB. The state of the art in survey analysis. In: Westlake A, et al, eds. *Survey and statistical computing*: Elsevier Science Publishers B.V; 1992.

[26] Heckman JJ, Borjas GJ. Does unemployment cause future unemployment? Definitions, Questions and Answers from a Continuous Time Model of Heterogeneity and State Dependence. *Econometrica*. 1980;47:247-83.

[27] Rubin D, Little R. *Statistical analysis with missing data*. New York: John Wiley and Sons; 2002.

[28] Shahtahmasebi S. *Statistical modelling of dependency in old age* [Ph.D], University of Wales, Bangor, North Wales; 1995.

[29] Shahtahmasebi S. Teenage Smoking: some problems in interpreting the evidence. *Int. J. Adolesc. Med. Health*. 2003;15(4):307-20.

[30] Shahtahmasebi S, Berridge D. Teenage smoking: A longitudinal analysis. *Int. J. Adolesc. Med. Health*. 2005;17(2):137-55.

[31] Cheshire J, Fox S, Kerswill P, Torgersen E. Ethnicity, friendship netwrok and social practice as the motor of dialect change:linguistic innovaiton in London. *Sociolinguistica*. 2008;22:1-24.

[32] Shahtahmasebi S, Wenger GC. Modelling the probability of survival in old age using GLIM. *CSPRD, University of Wales, Bangor, Gwynedd, UK* 1989.

[33] Shahtahmasebi S, Davies R, Wenger C. A longitudinal analysis of factors related to survival in old age. *The Gerontologist*. 1992;333:404-13.

[34] Pfeiffer E. Survival in old age. *Journal of the American Geriatric Society*. 1970;184:273-85.

[35] Harel Z. Discriminators between survivors and non-survivors among working class and living in the community. *The Gerontologist*. 1979;191:83-89.

[36] Abrams M. *People in their late sixties: A longitudinal survey of ageing, part I survivors and non-survivors*. Mitcham, Surrey: Age Concern Research Unit; 1983.

[37] Granick S, Patterson RD. *Human ageing II an eleven-year follow-up biometrical and behavioural study*: Rockville, MD, DHEW National Institute of Mental Health, Section of Mental Health of the Ageing;1971.

[38] Fox AJ, Goldblatt PO. *Longitudinal study socio-demographic mortality defferentials*. London: OPCS, HMSO; 1982.

[39] Hirdes J, Forbes W. Estimates of relative risk of mortality based on the Ontario longitudinal study of aging. *Canadian Journal of Aging*. 1989;8(3):222-37.

[40] Kaplan G, Barell V, Lusky A. Subjective state of health and survival in elderly adults. *J. of Gerontology*. 1988;434:s114-20.

[41] Kaplan GA, Camacho T. Perceived Health and Mortality: A Nine year Follow-up of the Human Population Laboratory Cohort. *American Journal of Epidemiology*. 1983;117:292-304.

[42] Kaplan GA, Seeman TE, Cohen RD, Knudsen LP, Guralnik J. Mortality Among the Elderly in the Alameda County Study: Behaviourial and Demographic Risk Factors. *American Journal of Public Health*. 1987;773:307-12.

[43] Jones DR. Heart Disease Morality Following Widowhood: Some Results From the OPCS Longitudinal Study. *Journal of Psychosomatic Research*. 1987;313:325-33.

[44] Mossey JM, Shapiro E. Self-rated health: A predictor of mortality among the elderly. *Am. J. of Pub. Health*. 1982;728:800-08.

[45] Palmore E. The Relative Importance of Social Factors in Predicting Longevity. In: Palmore E, Jeffers FC, eds. *Prediction of Lifespan*: Heath Lexington Books; 1971.

[46] Palmore E. Predictors of the Longevity Difference: A 25-Year Follow-up. *The Gerontologist*. 1982;226:513-18.

[47] Singer E, Garfinkel R, Cohen SM, et al. Mortality and Mental Health Evidence from the Medtown Manhattan Restudy. *Soc. Sci. Med*. 1976;10:517-25.

[48] Townsend P, Davidson N. *Inequalities in Health - The Black Report*. Suffolk: The Chaucer Press; 1982.

[49] Thompson LW, Breckenridge JN, Gallagher D, Peterson J. Effects of Bereavement on Self-Perceptions of Physical Health in Elderly Widows and Widowers. *J. of Gerontology*. 1984;393:309-14.

[50] Jagger C, Sutton CJ. Death after bereavement - Is the risk increased? *Statistics in Medicine*. 1991;10:395-404.

[51] Berkman LF, Syme SL. Social Networks, Host Resistance, and Mortality A Nine-Year Follow-up Study of Alameda County Residents. *American Journal of Epidemiology*. 1979;109:186-204.

[52] *Generalised Linear Interactive Modelling* [computer program]. Version 3.77. Oxford, U.K: NAG; 1987.

[53] Bishop YMM, Fienberg SE, Holland PW. *Discrete Multivariate Analysis- Theory and Practice*. London, England: The MIT press; 1988.

[54] McCullagh P. Regression models for ordinal data. *Journal of the Royal Statistical Society*. 1980;Series B 42:109-42.

[55] Davies RB. *A reappraisal of some simple statistical models*: Centre for Applied Statistics, Lancaster University;1984.

[56] Dykstra P, van Tilburg T, Gierveld J. Changes in older adult loneliness: Results from a seven-year longitudinal study. *Research on Aging.* 2005;27(6):725.

[57] Booth T, Bilson A. Wells of Loneliness? *Insight.* 1988(March).

[58] Wenger GC. Support Networks in Old Age: Constructing a Typology. In: Jefferys M, ed. *Growing Old in the Twentieth Century.* London: Routledge; 1989:166-85.

[59] Cox DR, Oakes D. *Analysis of Survival Data.* New York: Chapman and Hall; 1984.

[60] Kalbfleisch JD, Prentice RL. *The Statistical Analysis of Failure Time Data.* New York: Wiley; 1980.

[61] Lawless JF. *Statistical Models and Methods for Lifetime Data.* New York: Wiley; 1982.

[62] Version Mark 14. Oxford, UK: NAG ltd; 1990.

[63] Shahtahmasebi S. The application of instrumental variables in correcting model mis-specification in the analysis of longitudinal observational data. In: Friedl H, Berghold A, Kauermann G, eds. *Statistical Modelling*: 14th International Workshop on Statistical Modelling in Graz/Austria, 19-23 July; 1999.

[64] Sullivan MD. Maintaining good morale in old age. *West J. Med.* Oct 1997;167(4):276-84.

[65] Buntix F, Kestner A, Bergers J, Knottnerus JA. Is depression in elderly people followed by dementia? A retrospective cohort study based in general practice. *Age and Ageing.* 1996;25:231-33.

[66] Kay DW, Beamish P, Roth M. Old age mental disorder in Newcastle on Tyne: Part I, a study of prevalence. *Brit. J. Psychiat.* 1964;110:668.

[67] Orrell M, Bebbington P. Life events and senile dementia. *British Journal of Psychiatry.* 1995;166:613-20.

[68] Snowdon J, Lane F. The Botany survey: a longitudinal study of depression and cognitive impairment in an elderly population. *Int. J. Geriat. Psychiat.* 1995;10:349-58.

[69] Copeland JRM, Davidson IA, Dewey ME, et al. Alzheimer's disease, other dementias, depression and pseudo-dementia: prevalence, incidence and three-year outcome in Liverpool. *Brit. J. Psychiat.* 1992;161:230-39.

[70] Green BH, Copeland JRM, Dewey ME, Shrma V, Davidson IA. Factors associated with rcovery and recurrence of depression in older people: a prospective study. *Int. J. Geriat. Psychiat.* 1994;9:789-95.

[71] Iliffe S, Haines A, Gallivan S, Booroff A, Oldenberg E, Morgan P. Assessment of elderly people in general practice: 1. Social Circumstances and mental state. *British Journal of General Practice.* 1991;41:9-12.

[72] Macdonald A. Do general practicners 'miss' depression in elderly patients? *BMJ.* 1986;292:1365-67.

[73] Wattis JP. Difficulties in diagnosis of depression in the elderly. *Spectrum International.* 1995;XXXV:6-7.

[74] Waxman HM, Carner EA. Physician's recognition, diagnosis and treatment of mental disorders in elderly medical patients. *Gerontologist.* 1984;24(6):593-97.

[75] Parmalee PA, Katz IR, Lawton MP. The relation of pain to depression among institutionalised aged. *Journal of Gerontology.* 1991;46(1):15-21.

[76] Ventegodt S, Andersen NJ, Merrick J. Quality of Life Philosophy VI. The concepts. *TheScientificWorldJOURNAL.* 2003;3:1230-40.

[77] Ventegodt S, Andersen NJ, Merrick J. Quality of Life Philosophy I. Quality of life, happiness, and meaning in life. *TheScientificWorldJOURNAL.* 2003;3:1164-75.

[78] Ventegodt S, Henneberg E, Merrick J, Lindholt J. Validation of two global and generic quality of life questionnaires for population screening: SCREENQOL and SEQOL. *TheScientificWorldJOURNAL.* 2003;3:412-21.

[79] Ventegodt S, Hilden J, Merrick J. Measurement of Quality of Life I. A Methodological Framework. *TheScientificWorldJOURNAL.* 2003;3:950-61.

[80] Ventegodt S, Merrick J. Lifestyle, quality of life, and health. *TheScientificWorldJOURNAL.* 2003;3:811-25.

[81] Ventegodt S, Merrick J. Measurement of quality of life VII. Statistical Covariation and global quality of life data: the method of weight-modified linear regression. *TheScientificWorldJOURNAL.* 2003;3:1020-29.

[82] Ventegodt S, Merrick J, Andersen NJ. Quality of Life Theory I. The IQOL Theory: an integrative theory of the global quality of life concept. *TheScientificWorldJOURNAL.* 2003;3:1030-40.

[83] Ventegodt S, Merrick J, Andersen NJ. Measurement of Quality of Life II. From the philosophy of life to science. *The Scientifi WorldJOURNAL.* 2003;3:962-71.

[84] Ventegodt S, Merrick J, Andersen NJ. Quality of life as medicine: a pilot study of patients with chronic illness and pain. *TheScientificWorldJOURNAL.* 2003;3:520-32.

[85] Wenger GC, Davies R, Shahtahmasebi S. Morale in Old Age: Refining the Model. *International Journal of Geriatric Psychiatry.* 1995;10:933-43.

[86] Gibbons RD, Hedeker DR, Elkin I, Waternaux C, et al. Some conceptual and statistal issues in analysis of longitudinal psychiatric data: Application to the NIMH Treatment of Depression Collaborative Research Program dataset. *Archives of General Psychiatry.* 1993;50(9):739-50.

[87] Davics RB. From cross-sectional to longitudinal analysis. In: Dale A, Davies RB, eds. *Analysing social and political change: A casebook of methods.* London: Sage; 1994:20-40.

[88] Everitt BS. Analysis of longitudinal data: beyond MANOVA. *British Journal of Psychiatry.* 1998;172:7-10.

[89] Lawton MP. The Philadelphia Geriatric Centre Morale Scale a revision. *Journal of Gerontology.* 1975;30:85-89.

[90] Pfeiffer E. *The older American Resources Scale*, Duke University, North Carolina, U S A; 1975.

[91] Challis D, Knapp M. *An Examination of the PGC Morale Scale in an English Context*: PSSRV, University of Kent;1980.

[92] Liang J, Lawrence RH, Bollen KA. Age Differences in the Structure of the Philadelphia Geriatric Morale Scale. *Journal of Psychology and Aging.* 1986;11:27-33.

[93] Shahtahmasebi S, Davies R, Wenger C. Morale in old age: A cross-sectional analysis. *CSPRD, UCNW, Bangor, UK* 1991.

[94] Grundy EM, Bowling A. Household Transitions and Health among Elderly People: Analyses of Longitudinal Data from England and Wales. *Sociological Abstracts, Inc.* 1994.

[95] Grundy EMD. Socio-Demographic Variations in Rates of Movement into Institutions Among Elderly People in England and Wales: An Analysis of Linked Census and Mortality Data 1971-1985. *Population Studies.* 1992;46:65-84.

[96] Wenger GC. *Old people's health and experiences of the caring services - Account from rural communities in North Wales.* Vol 4: The Institute of human ageing, Liverpool University Press; 1988.

[97] Anderson TW, Hsiao C. Estimation of dynamic models with error components. *American Statistics Association.* 1981;76(375).

[98] Chamberlain G. Analysis of Covariance with Qualitative Data Review of Economic Studies. *XLVII.* 1980:225-38.

[99] Amemiya T. *Advanced econometrics*: Blackwell; 1985.

[100] Amemiya T, MaCurdy T. Instrumental variable estimation of an error- components model. *Econometrics.* 1986;544:869-80.

[101] *Variance Component Analysis VARCL* [computer program]. Lancaster: Centre for Applied Statistics, Lancaster University; 1986.

[102] Crouchley R, Berridge D. *Multivariate Generalized Linear Mixed Models Using R* London: Chapman and Hall; forthcoming.

[103] Crouchley R, Davies R. A comparison of population average and random effect models for the analysis of longitudinal count data with base-line information. *Journal of the Royal Statistical Society, Series A.* 1999;162:331-47.

[104] Crouchley R, Davies R. A comparison of GEE and random effects models for distinguishing heterogeneity, nonstationarity and state dependence in a collection of short binary event series. *Statistical Modelling.* 2001;1(271-285).

[105] Bohning D, Ekkehart DE, Schlattmann P, L. M, Kirchner U. The Zero-Inflated Poisson Model and the Decayed, Missing and Filled Teeth Index in Dental Epidemiology. *Journal of the Royal Statistical Society. Series A (Statistics in Society).* 1999;162:195-209.

[106] Goodman L. Statistical methods for the mover stayer model. *Journal of the American Statistical Association.* 1961;56:841-68.

[107] Singer B, Spillerman S. Some methodological issues in the analysis of longitudinal surveys. *Annals of Economic and Social Measurement.* 1976;5:447-74.

[108] Heckman JJ, Singer B. A method for minimizing the impact of distributional assumptions in econometric models of duration data. *Econometrica.* 1984;52:271-320.

[109] Davies R, Crouchley R. The Mover-Stayer Model Requiescat in Pace. *Sociological Methods and Research.* 1986;14:356-80.

[110] McGinnis R. A Stochastic model of social mobility. *American Sociological Review.* 1968;23:712-22.

[111] Heckman J. Micro data, heterogeneity and the evaluation of public policy: Nobel lecture. *Journal of Political Economy.* 2001;109(673-748).

[112] Heckman J. The incidental parameters problem and the problem of initial conditions in estimating a discrete time-discrete data stochastic process. In: Manski C, McFadden D, eds. *Structural Analysis of Discrete Data with Econometric Applications.* Cambridge, Mass: MIT press; 1981.

[113] Bhargava A, Sargan J. Estimating dynamic random effects models from panel data covering short time periods. *Econometrica.* 1983;51:1635-57.

[114] Alfò M, Aitkin M. Variance component models for longitudinal count data with baseline information: epilepsy data revisited. *Statistics and Computing.* 2006;16:231-38.

[115] Wooldridge J. Simple solutions to the initial conditions problem in dynamic, nonlinear panel data models with unobserved heterogeneity. *Journal of Applied Econometrics.* 2005;20:39-54.

[116] Kazemi I, Crouchley R. Modelling the initial conditions in dynamic regression models of panel data with random effects. In: Baltagi B, ed. *Panel Data Econometrics, theoretical Contributions and Empirical Applications.* Amsterdam, Netherlands: Elsevier; 2006.

[117] Stewart M. The interrelated dynamics of unemployment and low-wage employment. *Journal of Applied Econometrics.* 2007;22(511-531).

[118] Hsiao C. *Analysis of Panel Data.* Vol, Cambridge University Press, Cambridge. Cambridge: Cambridge University Press; 1986.

[119] Likert R. A technique for the measurement of attitudes. *Archives of Psychology* 1932;140:1-55.

[120] Bolling K. *Smoking among secondary school children in England in 1993. An enquiry carried out by Social Survey Division of OPCS on behalf of the Department of Health*: OPCS. Social Survey Division London:HMSO;1994.

[121] Goddard E. *Why children start smoking. An enquiry carried out by the Social Survey Division of OPCS on behalf of the Department of Health*: OPCS, Social Survey Division London:HMSO;1990.

[122] Hine C. *Report on stopping or reducing smoking: issues for Health Authorities*: Health Care Evaluation Unit. Department of Epidemiology and Public Health Medicine. University of Bristol;1992.

[123] Jensen EJ, Overgaard E. Investigation of Smoking Habits among 14-17-year-old Boarding School Pupils: Factors which influence Smoking Status. *Public Health.* 1993;107:117-23.

[124] Lader D, Matheson J. *Smoking among secondary school children in 1990. An enquiry carried out by Social Survey Division of OPCS on behalf of the Department of Health, the Welsh Office and the Scottish Office Home and Health Department*: OPCS, Social Survey Division. London:HMSO;1991.

[125] Pletcher JR, Schwarz DF. Current concepts in adolescent smoking. *Curr. Opin. Pediatr.* Oct 2000;12(5):444-9.

[126] Tyas SL, Pederson LL. Psychosocial factors related to adolescent smoking: a critical review of the literature. *Tob. Control.* Winter 1998;7(4):409-20.

[127] Sussman SC, Dent W. Group self-identification and adolescent cigarette smoking: a 1-year prospective study. *J. Abnorm. Psychol.* 1994;103(3):576-80.

[128] Murphy NT, Price CJ. The influence of self-esteem, parental smoking and living in tobacco production region on adolescent smoking behaviour. *J. Sch. Health.* 1988;58(10):401-5.

[129] Moore S, Gullone E. Predicting adolescent risk behaviour using a personalized cost-benefit analysis. *J. Youth Adolesc.* 1996;25(3):343-59.

[130] Parsons JT, Siegel AW, Cousins JH. Late adolescent risk-taking: effect of perceived benefits and perceived risks on behavioural intentions and behavioural change. *J. Adolesc.* 1997;20:381-92.

[131] Smith AMA, Rosenthal DA. Adolescents' perceptions of their risk environment. *J. Adolesc.* 1995;18:229-45.

[132] McNeill AD, Jarvis M, West R. Subjective effects of cigarette smoking in adolescents. *Psychopharmacology-(Berl).* 1987;92(1):115-7.

[133] Upadhyaya HP, Deas D, Brady KT, Kruesi M. Cigarette smoking and psychiatric comorbidity in children and adolescents. *Journal of the American Academy of Child and Adolescent Psychiatry.* Nov 2002;41(11):1294-305.

[134] Shek DT. Family environment and adolescent psychological well-being, school adjustment, and problem behaviour: a pioneer study in a Chinese context. *J. Genet. Psychol.* 1997;158(1):113-28.

[135] Clayton S. Gender differences in psychosocial determinants of adolescent smoking. *J. Sch. Health.* 1991;61(3):115-20.

[136] Paavola M, Vartianian E, Puska P. Predicting adult smoking: the influence of smoking during adolescence and smoking among friends and family. *Health Educ. Res.* 1996;11(3):309-15.

[137] Soldz S, Cui X. Pathways through adolescent smoking: a 7-year longitudinal grouping analysis. *Health Psychol.* Sep 2002;21(5):495-504.

[138] McNeill AD. The development of dependence on smoking in children. *Psychopharmacology-(Berl).* 1991;92(1):115-7.

[139] Bell R, Pavis S, Amos A, Cunningham-Burley S. Continuities and changes: teenage smoking and occupational transition. *J. Adolesc.* Oct 1999;22(5):683-94.

[140] Carlin JB, Wolfe R, Coffey C, Patton GC. Analysis of binary outcomes in longitudinal studies using weighted estimating equations and discrete-time survival methods: prevalence and incidence of smoking in an adolescent cohort. *Stat. Med..* Oct 15 1999;18(19):2655-79.

[141] Sashegyi AI, Brown KS, Farrell PJ. Application of a generalized random effects regression model for cluster-correlated longitudinal data to a school-based smoking prevention trial. *Am. J. Epidemiol.* Dec 15 2000;152(12):1192-200.

[142] Higgins A, Conner M. Understanding adolescent smoking: the role of the Theory of Planned Behaviour and implementation intentions. *Psychology, Health and Medicine.* 2003;8(2):173-86.

[143] **Lawlor D, O'Callaghan J, AA. M, et al. Early life predictors** of adolescent smoking: findings from the Mater-University study of pregnancy and its outcomes. *Paediatric and Perinatal Epidemiology.* 2005;19:377-87.

[144] Shahtahmasebi S. Teenage smoking: researching behaviour. *Int. J. of Psychology Research.* 2007;2(1/2).

[145] Shahtahmasebi S. Teenage smoking: what are the main issues? In: Lapointe MM, ed. *Adolescent Smoking and Health Research.* New York: Nova Sci; 2007:91-102.

[146] Shahtahmasebi S. Teenage smoking: longitudinal vs. cross-sectional modeling. In: Grenell RS, ed. *Adolescent Behaviour Research Studies.* New York: Nova Sci; 2007:77-107.

[147] Balding J. *Young People in 1991*: Schools Health Education Unit, University of Exeter;1992.

[148] Davies R, Flowerdew R. Modelling Migration Careers Using Data from a British Survey. *Geographical Analysis.* 1992;24:35-57.

[149] Davies R, Pickles A. Accounting for omitted variables in a discrete time panel data of residual mobility. *Quality and Quantity.* 1986;20:219-33.

[150] Braverman MT. Research on resilience and its implications for tobacco prevention. *Nicotine Tob. Res.* 1999(1 Suppl 1):S67-72.

[151] Charlton A. The Brigantia Smoking Survey: a general review. Public Education About Cancer. *UICC Technical Report Series.* 1984;77:92-102.

[152] Eiser J, Morgan M, Gammage P, Gray E. Adolescent smoking: attitudes, norms and parental influences. *British Journal of Soc. Physio.* 1989;28:193-202.

[153] US Department of Health and Human Services. *Preventing Tobacco Use Among Young People. A Report of the Surgeon General*: Public Health Service, Centers for Disease Control and Prevention, National Center for Chronic Disease Prevention and Health Promotion, Office on Smoking and Health;1994.

[154] MacFadyen L, Hastings G, Mackintosh A. Cross sectional study of young people's awareness of and involvement with tobacco marketing. *BMJ.* 2001;3(322):513-7.

[155] Norton EC, Lindrooth RC, Ennett ST. How measures of perception from survey data lead to inconsistent regression results: evidence from adolescent and peer substance use. *Health Econ.* Feb 2003;12(2):139-48.

[156] Flay BR, Hu FB, Siddiqui O, et al. Differential influence of parental smoking and friends' smoking on adolescent initiation and escalation of smoking. *Journal of Health and Social Behavior.* 1994;35(3):248-65.

[157] Duffy JC, ed *Alcohol and illness: the epidemiological view point.* Edinburgh: Edinburgh University Press; 1992. Health and Society.

[158] Marcus P, Newman B, Millikan R, Moorman P, Baird D, Qaqish B. The associations of adolescent cigarette smoking, alcoholic beverage consumption, environmental tobacco smoke, and ionizing radiation with subsequent breast cancer risk (United States). *Cancer Causes and Control.* 2000;11(3):271-78.

[159] Kosterman R. The dynamics of alcohol and marijuana initiation: patterns and predictors of first use in adolescence. *American Journal of Public Health.* Vol 90. Am Public Health Assoc; 2000:360-66.

[160] Rashad I, Kaestner R. Teenage sex, drugs and alcohol use: problems identifying the cause of risky behaviors. *Journal of Health Economics.* 2004;23(3):493-503.

[161] Weinberg N, Rahdert E, Colliver J, Glantz M. Adolescent substance abuse: a review of the past 10 years. *Journal of the American Academy of Child and Adolescent Psychiatry.* 1998;37(3):252-61.

[162] Peterson P, Hawkins J, Abbott R, Catalano R. Disentangling the Effects of Parental Drinking, Family Management, and Parental Alcohol Norms on Current Drinking by Black and White Adolescents. *Journal of Research on Adolescence.* 1994;4(2):203-27.

[163] White HR, McMorris BJ, Catalano RF, Fleming CB, Haggerty KP, Abbott RD. Increases in alcohol and marijuana use during the transition out of high school into emerging adulthood: The effects of leaving home, going to college, and high school protective factors. *J. Stud. Alcohol.* Nov 2006;67(6):810-22.

[164] Wilks J, Callan V, Austin D. Parent, Peer and Personal Determinants of Adolescent Drinking. *Addiction.* 1989;84(6):619-30.

[165] Dawson DA, Grant BF, Li TK. Impact of age at first drink on stress-reactive drinking. *Alcohol Clin. Exp. Res.* Jan 2007;31(1):69-77.

[166] de Visser RO, Rissel CE, Smith AM, Richters J. Sociodemographic correlates of selected health risk behaviors in a representative sample of Australian young people. *Int. J. Behav. Med.* 2006;13(2):153-62.

[167] Grucza RA, Bierut LJ. Cigarette smoking and the risk for alcohol use disorders among adolescent drinkers. *Alcohol Clin. Exp. Res.* Dec 2006;30(12):2046-54.

[168] Loury S, Kulbok P. Correlates of alcohol and tobacco use among Mexican immigrants in rural North Carolina. *Fam. Community Health.* Jul-Sep 2007;30(3):247-56.

[169] Agrawal A, Grant JD, Waldron M, et al. Risk for initiation of substance use as a function of age of onset of cigarette, alcohol and cannabis use: findings in a Midwestern female twin cohort. *Prev. Med.* Aug 2006;43(2):125-8.

[170] Amonini C, Donovan RJ. The relationship between youth's moral and legal perceptions of alcohol, tobacco and marijuana and use of these substances. *Health Educ. Res.* Apr 2006;21(2):276-86.

[171] Atkin C. Effects of televised alcohol messages on teenage drinking patterns. *J. Adolesc. Health Care.* 1990;11(1):10-24.

[172] Bates M, Labouvie E. Adolescent risk factors and the prediction of persistent alcohol and drug use into adulthood. *Alcohol Clin. Exp. Res.* 1997;21(5):944-50.

[173] Chuang YC, Ennett ST, Bauman KE, Foshee VA. Neighborhood influences on adolescent cigarette and alcohol use: mediating effects through parent and peer behaviors. *J. Health Soc. Behav.* Jun 2005;46(2):187-204.

[174] Engels RC, Scholte RH, van Lieshout CF, de Kemp R, Overbeek G. Peer group reputation and smoking and alcohol consumption in early adolescence. *Addict. Behav.* Mar 2006;31(3):440-9.

[175] Orlando M, Tucker JS, Ellickson PL, Klein DJ. Concurrent use of alcohol and cigarettes from adolescence to young adulthood: an examination of developmental trajectories and outcomes. *Subst. Use Misuse.* 2005;40(8):1051-69.

[176] Blum R. The effects of race/ethnicity, income, and family structure on adolescent risk behaviors. *Am. J. Public Health.* 2000;90(12):1879-84.

[177] Heath A, Madden P, Grant J, McLaughlin T, Todorov A, Bucholz K. Resiliency factors protecting against teenage alcohol use and smoking: influences of religion, religious involvement and values, and ethnicity in the Missouri Adolescent Female Twin Study. *Twin Research and Human Genetics.* 1999;2(2):145-55.

[178] Rose R, Dick D, Viken R, Kaprio J. Gene-Environment Interaction in Patterns of Adolescent Drinking: Regional Residency Moderates Longitudinal Influences on Alcohol Use. *Alcohol Clin. Exp. Res.* 2001;25(5):637.

[179] Bonomo Y, Bowes G, Coffey C, Carlin J, Patton G. Teenage drinking and the onset of alcohol dependence: a cohort study over seven years. *Addiction.* 2004;99(12):1520.

[180] Cassidy B, Shahtahmasebi S. Literacy and ICT: I. Young People with Learning Difficulties. *Int. J. of Medical and Biological Frontiers.* 2009;15(1/2):forthcoming.

[181] Royal College of Physicians. *Smoking and the Young.* London1992.

[182] Stuart A. *The idea of sampling.* High Wycombe: Charles Griffin and Company Ltd; 1984.

[183] Caldock K. *Domiciliary Services and dependency A Meaningful relationship?*: CSPRD, University of Wales, Bangor;1990.

[184] Wenger GC. Surviving in the Community: some demographic and social factors. *CSPRD, University of Bangor, UK* 1984.

[185] Wenger GC. *Support networks: change and stability second report of a follow-up study of old elderly people in North Wales*: CSPRD, University of Bangor, UK;1987.

[186] Wenger GC. *Relationships in old age - inside support networks: third report of a follow-up study of old elderly people in North Wales*: CSPRD, University of Bangor, UK;1987.

[187] *Software for Analysis of Binary Recurrent Events (SABRE): A guide for users* [computer program]. Lancaster: Centre for Applied Statistics, Lancaster University; 1990. www.SABRE.lancs.ac.uk.

APPENDIX I – LIST OF EXPLANATORY VARIABLES

A. LIST OF VARIABLES USED IN SURVIVAL ANALYSIS SECTIONS (CHAPTER 2)

Explanatory variable	Description/type
Age	continuous
Sex	male, female
Income	under £60; £60-99; over £100 per week
Social class	I/II (middle class), III (skilled working class), IV/V (semi and unskilled working class)
Home tenure	owner occupier, rented accommodation, other (including living with relatives, caravan and lodgings)
Ethnicity	Welsh, half Welsh, English, British, other
Marital status	single, married, widowed/divorce/separated
Number of children	counts
Arrival age in community	long term resident (in community before 40 years of age); middle aged mover (arrived in community aged 40-60); retirement mover (those who moved short distances after age 60); retirement migrant (those who moved more than 50 miles after age 60)
Household composition	lives alone, with spouse, with others (including children, other relatives)
Relative seen most often	children; siblings; nephew/niece/cousin; other
Frequency of contact with family	every day; at most once a week; at least once a month; less than once a month
Number in support network	*network size* [2]: small, medium, large, missing
Network type	family dependent; locally integrated; local self-contained; wider community focussed; private restricted [58]
Hours spent alone	up to 6 hours; more than 6 hours
Isolation measure	combination of 7 variables indicating contact/access to family, friends/neighbours and transport/telephone, see [2]
Loneliness measure	
Morale	low, medium, high (see Chapter 3)
Self-assessed loneliness	lonely, not lonely
Worry over bills	worry, do not worry
Self-assessed state of health	excellent/good, allright for age, fair, poor
Health limited activities	yes (limited activity due to a health condition), no
Visit from doctor	yes (visited by doctor in the last 6 months prior to interview), no
Visit from district nurse	yes (visited by district nurse in the last 6 months prior to interview), no
Visit from home help	yes (visited by home-help in the last 6 months prior to interview), no
Visit from private home help	yes (visited by private home-help in the last 6 months prior to interview), no
Cumulative Pfeiffer score	combination of the 5 Pfeiffer scores

B. LIST OF VARIABLES USED IN THE ANALYSIS OF MORALE IN OLD AGE (CHAPTER 3)

Explanatory variable	Description/type
Age	continuous
Sex	male, female
Income	under £60; £60-99; over £100 per week
Social class	I/II (middle class), III (skilled working class), IV/V (semi and unskilled working class)
Home tenure	owner occupier, rented accommodation, other (including living relatives, caravan and lodgings)
Ethnicity	Welsh, half Welsh, English, British, other (alternatively: Welsh, non-Welsh)
Marital status	single, married, widowed/divorce/separated
Number of children	counts
Arrival age in community	long term resident (in community before 40 years of age); middle aged mover (arrived in community aged 40-60); retirement mover (those who moved short distances after age 60); retirement migrant (those who moved more than 50 miles after age 60)
Relative seen most often	children; siblings; nephew/niece/cousin; other
Frequency of contact with family	every day; at most once a week; at least once a month; less than once a month
Who cares when ill	spouse, relative in/out of house, friend/neighbour, other, no one/don't know/missing
change in marital status	no change, lost spouse, married
Number of years widowed	counts
Housebound	yes, no
Self-assessed state of health	excellent/good, allright for age, fair, poor
Health limited activities	yes (limited activity due to a health condition), no
Household composition	lives alone, with spouse, with others (including children, other relatives)
Hours spent alone	0-3 hours per day, 3-9 hours per day, 9+ hours perday
Has close relatives	yes, no
Visit relatives	at least weekly, at least 6 times per year, less often, no relatives/never
Has telephone	yes, no
Nearest neighbour	next door, across road/50-100 yards away, 100+ yards away
Isolation measure	combination of 7 variables indicating contact/access to family, friends/neighbours and transport/telephone, see [2]
Network type	family dependent; locally integrated; local self-contained; wider community focussed; private restricted [58]
People available to do favours	yes, no, never ask favours
Presence of real friends in community	yes, no
Wish for more friends	yes, no
Confidant	no-one, spouse, other
Self-assessed loneliness	never, rarely, sometimes, often/always
Pfeiffer social rating scale	categorical; 1= socially active,..., 5=socially inactive
Pfeiffer mental health rating scale	categorical; 1= socially active,..., 5=socially inactive
Pfeiffer physical health rating scale	categorical; 1= socially active,..., 5=socially inactive
Pfeiffer activities of daily living scale	categorical; 1= socially active,..., 5=socially inactive
Pfeiffer economic resources rating scale	categorical; 1= socially active,..., 5=socially inactive
Cumulative Pfeiffer score	combination of the above 5 ratings (see [96, 183])

C. FURTHER DETAILS OF EXPLANATORY VARIABLES LISTED IN SECTIONS A AND B

Home tenure:- Tenants tend to have a lower survival rate probably due to *class, income* or *education* differences. There are no measures of educational levels in the North Wales data set, but there are measures of *social class, types of accommodation* and *income*. Type of accommodation (*home tenure*) is included as a proxy variable for some of the socio-economic effects not fully represented by the social class and income measures. Three types of accommodation were distinguished: *owner occupiers, tenants* (those in rented accommodation) and *others* (those who lived with others- with relatives/friends or in lodgings).

Cumulative Pfeiffer score:- the Pfeiffer scales were only available for 1983 and 1987. From these scales, a cumulative score was calculated (see [183]) as a more objective assessment of dependency than the subjective self-assessed dependency.

Morale, loneliness and isolation:- the Philadelphia Geriatric Centre morale scale [89], self-assessed loneliness, a loneliness measure (an aggregate of 8 variables indicating feelings of loneliness, see [184]), and an isolation measure (an aggregate of 10 variables indicating isolation in terms of access to telephone, transport, nearest neighbour and so on, see [184]) were included in the list. The basic concern is to investigate the relationship between these socio-psychological variables and survival of the elderly.

Arrival age in community:- Although this is classified as a demographic variable, it may be seen as a proxy for levels and availability of informal help within the community. It is postulated that those who arrived in the community before or during childrearing age are more likely to have local kin, friends and neighbours networks than those who arrived in middle or old age. Thus, it is of interest to explore variations in survival, if any, between those who have more access to kin/help in the face of growing dependency and those who have little or no established supportive network. This concern also leads to the inclusion of a new variable *network type* which deals with the nature of supportive networks as they relate to *distinctive* needs and requirements of the elderly person (see Section D).

D. NETWORK TYPE

Network type:- The network typology was developed by Wenger [58, 185, 186]. In summary, the typology consists of five categories:

1. *The family dependent support network* has a primary focus on nearby kin ties, close family relationships and few peripheral friends and neighbours. It is often based on a shared household with adult children, sister(s) or brother(s), or very near separate households. Most commonly the old person relies primarily on a daughter.
2. *The locally integrated support network* includes close relationships with local family, friends and neighbours. Many friends are also neighbours. Usually based on long-term residence and active community involvement in the present or recent past.
3. *The local self-contained support network* typically has arms-length relationships or infrequent contact, with at least one relative living in the same or adjacent community, usually a sibling, niece or nephew. Reliance is focussed on neighbours but respondents with this type of network adopt a household-focussed lifestyle and community involvement, if any, tends to be very low key.
4. *The wider community-focussed support network* is typified by active relationships with distant relatives, usually children, high salience of friends and few neighbours. Distinction between friends and neighbours is maintained. Respondents with this type of network are generally involved in community voluntary organizations. Absence of local kin is common. This network is commonly a middle-class adaptation.

5. *The private restricted support network* is associated with absence of local kin, other than in some cases a spouse; minimal contact with neighbours, no nearby local friends and lack of wider community contacts or involvements.

APPENDIX II – BINARY RESPONSE MODEL

I. Probability of Survival (Success)

To fit a regression model to a binary response variable (coded 1/0 to indicate yes/no or success/failure) the data need to be transformed. Generally a suitable transformation is the logit with the probability of 'success' (1) given by:

$$\text{logit}\{p(y_i = 1) = \log\{\frac{p(y_i = 1)}{p(y_i = 0)}\} = \beta x_i$$

or

$$p(y_i) = \frac{\exp(\beta x_i)}{1 + \exp(\beta x_i)}$$

Where y_i is the response variable, x_i is the explanatory variable, β is the coefficient of x_i.

II. Calculating Non-Survival

We can estimate the death (failure) rate from the sample which is about 40% between 1979 and 1987 (about 20% between 1979 and 1983). We calculate the value of linear predictor $\varphi = x\beta$ as follows:

$$p(y = 0; death) = \frac{1}{1 + \exp(\phi)} = 0.4 \quad (@\ 40\%)$$

$$1 = 0.4 + 0.4 * \exp(\phi) \quad i.e. \quad \exp(\phi) = \frac{0.6}{0.4} = 1.5$$

Now to calculate what difference it would make to an individual with estimated i^{th} parameter (e.g. -1.24 for an individual in poor state of health from Table 2.4), we write

$$p = \frac{1}{1+\exp(\phi+\beta_i)} = \frac{1}{1+1.5\exp(\beta_i)} = \frac{1}{1+1.5\exp(-1.24)} = 0.75$$

Thus, those who claimed to be in a fair or poor state of health are 0.75 times as likely to survive as those who claimed to be in a good state of health.

APPENDIX III – MULTINOMIAL RESPONSE MODEL

The response Y_i may take a value between 1 and k (k=3 for the exercise in Section 2.5), and the probability that the ith individual takes a value Y_i=m (1<=m<=k), is given by (see also [23]):

$$p(y_i = m \mid x_i) = \frac{\exp(\beta x_i)}{\sum_{j=1}^{k}\exp(\beta x_j)}$$

Such a model could be operationalized using any standard statistical software such as GLIM4, LIMDEP, NLOGIT, R, SABRE, SAS, STATA, S+.

Given that we assumed the response is ordered, then the multinomial model can be re-specified as follows in (1), (2) and (3) (see [23, 55]):

$$p_{i1} = \frac{\exp(-\alpha_1 + \beta x_i)}{1+\exp(-\alpha_1 + \beta x_i)} \tag{1}$$

$$p_{i2} = \frac{\exp(-\alpha_2 + \beta x_i)}{1+\exp(-\alpha_2 + \beta x_i)} - p_{i1} \tag{2}$$

$$p_{i3} = 1 - p_{i2} - p_{i1} \tag{3}$$

with individual i making the following contribution to the likelihood function:

$$L_i = \{[p_{i1}]^w \cdot [p_{i2}]^z \cdot [p_{i3}]^{(1-w)(1-z)}\}$$

where w=1 if individual I is a survivor and in the community; =0 otherwise, and z=1 if the same individual is a survivor and in residential care; =0 otherwise.

The 'latent' variable in this formulation is given by: $y=\beta^T x_i + \varepsilon_i$, where ε_i has logistic distribution: if $y_i > \alpha_1$ there is survival in the community, if $\alpha_2 < y_i \leq \alpha_1$ there is entry into residential care, and if $y_i \leq \alpha_2$ then death. The constant terms α_1 and α_2 within the linear predictor may be interpreted as 'boundary' parameters. This is demonstrated in Figure 2.2 (Section 2.5.2). Other ordinal specifications are possible [23], but the approach adopted here has the advantage of needing only a single linear predictor βx_i (see also [55]).

APPENDIX IV – DURATION DEPENDENCE MODEL

The duration T survived by an elderly person during the study may be characterized by the survivor function, which implies that the probability that an elderly person dies within the interval [t, t+δt] is given by its probability density function:

$$f(t) = p(t < T < t+\delta t)/\delta t$$

i.e. the probability that an individual dies in the interval [t,t+δt]. Therefore, the probability that the individual in the study dies by time t is given by the cumulative distribution function F(t):

$$F(t) = p(T \leq t) = \int_{x=0}^{t} f(x)dx$$

The probability that the individual has survived beyond t is given by the survivor function S(t):

$$S(t) = p(T > t) = \int_{x=t}^{\infty} f(x)dx$$

i.e. S(t)=1-F(t).

A useful feature of survival analysis is the concept of a hazard function h(t), which is the instantaneous rate of failure at time t:

$$h(t) = \lim_{\delta t \to 0} \frac{\Pr(t < T \leq t+\delta t \mid T > t)}{\delta t} = \frac{f(t)}{[1-F(t)]} = \frac{f(t)}{S(t)}$$

A probability distribution for survival can be specified equivalently by its density function, survivor function or hazard function. In practice, it is often more convenient and useful to specify the probability distribution by its hazard, facilitating model formulation and model interpretation. Detailed accounts of and discussion on survival analysis can be found in numerous statistical text books, notably [24, 59-61].

Due to the monotone increasing mortality rate in old age, the relationships between the various explanatory variables and survival can be investigated routinely within a conventional proportional hazards model using a Weibull specification for the temporal variation in the hazard (mortality) rate, as follows:

$$h(t) = \lambda \gamma t^{\gamma-1}$$

where λ is a function of the explanatory variables and for $\gamma=1$ the hazard is constant, $\gamma<1$ the hazard is decreasing, and $\gamma>1$ the hazard is increasing. An alternative specification which is often used for modelling human survival is the Gompertz, given by

$$h(t) = \lambda \exp(\alpha t)$$

This specification can also be investigated routinely. It was found to give very similar results for the explanatory variables but with a rather worse fit to the data (i.e. the log-likelihood was lower).

Appendix V – A Sufficient Statistic for a Binary Response

Reconsider the logistic probability for a binary response variable at time t (year=1983):

$$p(y_i = 1) = \frac{\exp(\beta x_{it})}{1+\exp(\beta x_{it})}$$

Similarly, the logistic probability for time t+1(=1987) is:

$$p(y_{it} = 1) = \frac{\exp(\beta x_{it+1})}{1+\exp(\beta x_{it+1})}$$

The probability, conditional on a sufficient statistic $y_{t+1}+y_t=1$, is given by:

$$p(S| y_{it+1} + y_{it} = 1) = \frac{\exp(x_{it+1} - x_{it})\beta}{1+\exp(x_{it+1} - x_{it})\beta}$$

where S is the observed sequence of outcomes({0,1} or {1,0}). Note that inference is based only on those individualsme status has changed e.g. from not lonely to lonely (0 to 1) and vice versa. This model may be fitted routinely using any standard statistical software such as GLIM4, LIMDEP, NLOGIT, S+, SABRE, SAS, STATA.

Appendix VI – Marginal Likelihood Method for a Continuous Response

Consider the model in equation (3.2) (Section 3.8) again:

$$y_{it} = \beta_0 + \beta x_{it} + \theta_i + \varepsilon_{it}$$

where the θs are the time-constant individual-specific errors and ε is the i.i.d. error term. To operationalise the model, the θs are eliminated by integrating them out of the likelihood. The likelihood is based on the probability or density unconditional on θ, given by (using the same notation as in Section 3.8):

$$f(S_i | \varphi; x_i) = \int f(S_i | \beta; x_i; \theta) f(\theta) d\theta$$

where $f(\theta)$ is the probability density function of θ, and the parameter vector φ consists of β and the parameters of $f(\theta)$. Therefore each case contributes to the likelihood:

$$L_i(\varphi) = \int L_i(\beta, \theta) df(\theta)$$

For a sample of N individuals (with up to T observations on each individual), the integrated or marginal log-likelihood is thus given by:

$$l = \sum_{i=1}^{N} \log L_i(\varepsilon) = \sum_{i=1}^{N} \log[f(S_i | \varphi; x_i)]$$

The integration will lead to the elimination of the nuisance terms θ from the model [16]. The individual-specific term θ_i and the i.i.d. error term ε_{it} (between intervals) are assumed to be normally distributed with zero mean and unknown variances σ_θ^2 and σ_ε^2, respectively, and zero covariances. It can be deduced that the intra-individual correlation is given by (see [12]):

$$R^2 = \frac{(\sigma_\theta)^2}{(\sigma_\theta)^2 + (\sigma_\varepsilon)^2}$$

APPENDIX VII – MARGINAL LIKELIHOOD METHOD FOR A BINARY RESPONSE

Reconsider the logistic model:

$$p(y_{it} = 1) = \frac{\exp(\beta x_{it})}{1 + \exp(\beta x_{it})}$$

Now let θ be the individual-specific term used in order to account for omitted variables (residual heterogeneity). Then we can re-write the logistic model to include explicitly this effect θ for individual i at time t:

$$p(y_{it} = 1) = \frac{\exp(\beta x_{it} + \theta_i)}{1 + \exp(\beta x_{it} + \theta_i)}$$

with contribution to the likelihood function of:

$$L_i = \frac{[\exp(\beta e_{it} + \theta_i)]^{y_{it}}}{1 + \exp(\beta x_{it} + \theta_i)}$$

The integrated likelihood for individual i is:

$$L_i = \int [\prod_{t=1}^{T_i} \frac{[e^{\beta x_{it} + \theta_i}]^{y_{it}}}{1 + e^{\beta x_{it} + \theta_i}}] f(\theta) d\theta$$

where T_i is the number of time points and $f(\theta)$ is the probability density function (mixing distribution) of θ, which is assumed to be normal, in which case the marginal/integrated likelihood may be evaluated using Gaussian quadrature (see also [187]).

APPENDIX VIII – ERRORS IN VARIABLES AND INSTRUMENTAL VARIABLES

Consider a continuous outcome y which may be measured with a set of observable explanatory variables {x} and unobservable variable ε:

$$y_i = \beta_0 + \beta x_i + \varepsilon_i . \qquad (4)$$

where $\{\varepsilon\}$ are i.i.d. random errors. In addition to the regression error, some of the observed x's may be subject to measurement error. For example, surveys which report measurements based on perceptions, attitudes and self-assessed characteristics give rise to such errors. Taking this into account, the above equation may be re-written as:

$$s_i = s'_i + \xi_i$$

Thus the true model that we wish to fit is given by:

$$y_i = \beta_0 + \beta x_i + \alpha(s_i - \xi_i) + \varepsilon_i \qquad (5)$$

where {s} are the observed values of the explanatory variables with measurement error ξ, {s'} are the 'true' values, and ε is the i.i.d. error term. However, ξ is unobserved and model (5) cannot be estimated. Generally, the following model in is fitted to data:

$$y_i = \beta_0 + \beta x_i + \alpha s_i + (\varepsilon_i - \alpha \xi_i) \qquad (6)$$

which is the same as model (4). It can be seen that the {s} are not independent of the error in model (6). This specification error is known as the 'error in variables'. The solution to this problem is the use of instrumental variables (see e.g. [19, 97]) where the variable(s) which is correlated with the error term is replaced by another variable which is known to be highly correlated with it, but has no association with the random error component. Such replacement variables are termed *instrumental* variables. Generally, in model 6, only the 'error free' {x} in the equation and those explanatory variables outside the model, but which may be available, may be used as instruments for the offending variables {s}. The {s} cannot be used since they are correlated with the error term (see [19]). To fit this model, we use the instrumental variables estimator [19, 97, 99, 100]:

$$\bar{\beta} = (z'x)^{-1} z'y$$

where z is the matrix containing the instrumental variable in its first column, and the explanatory variables in the remaining columns. In effect, for one variable, this is a two-stage least squares estimation process where predicted values from a regression of the problematic variable (past behaviour effect) on the instrument variable(s) is used to fit the model (3.7, Sub-section 3.8.2.2). There are computer packages that can handle such problems, for example, HUMMER (see [19]), R, SAS, Shazam, STATA and Time Series Processor (TSP),. For this exercise, TSP and HUMMER were used and produced similar results.

APPENDIX IX – CONTROLLING FOR TIME-VARIANT OMITTED VARIABLES

We could conceptualise a 'variance component' model to account explicitly for the time-variant omitted variables as follows:

$$y_{it} = \beta_0 + \beta x_{it} + \zeta_{it}$$

$$y_{it} = \beta_0 + \beta x_{it} + \theta_i + \xi_{it} + \varepsilon_{it} \tag{7}$$

where $\zeta = \theta + \xi + \varepsilon$; θ is the time-constant omitted heterogeneity, ξ is the time-variant omitted variable, and ε is i.i.d. random error. Similarly, for the next time point (t+1), we could write:

$$y_{it+1} = \beta_0 + \beta x_{it+1} + \theta_i + \xi_{it+1} + \varepsilon_{it+1} \tag{8}$$

It is *not* possible to operationalise this model using the conditional or integrated likelihood methods. Other methods will be computationally labour intensive and further assumptions about the mixing distribution will have to be made. Again, a pragmatic approach is required.

Recall the steps we took in the analysis of morale (Sub-sections 3.8.2.1 to 3.8.2.4). First, to improve the cross-sectional analysis, we distinguished between objective and subjective explanatory variables. Second, objective variables were those whose values could be verified independently, such as age and sex, and subjectively measured variables were those reported by the respondents, such as self-assessed health and loneliness. Therefore, such subjective variables carry measurement error. Third, in order to resolve specification problems with measurement error, we used instrumental variables. We can assume objective variables to be **'error' free and subjective variables** to be those subject to measurement error. We rewrite equation (8) to reflect this information:

$$y_{it} = \beta_0 + \beta x_{it} + \alpha s_{it} + \theta_i + \varepsilon_{it} \tag{9}$$

where $\{s\}$ are subjective explanatory variables, $\{x\}$ are objective explanatory variables, and $\{\theta\}$ and $\{\varepsilon\}$ are, as defined previously, the nuisance parameters. However, subjective variables themselves may be outcome variables. For example, the variable 'self-assessed' **health, say, may be the individuals'** own observed 'objective' or 'true' state of health plus some unobserved variables (e.g. the 'feel good' factor):

$$s = s' + \xi$$

where s is the observed value of the subjective variable, $\{s'\}$ is an individual's 'true' value and ξ is the i.i.d. unobserved error term. Thus, equation (9) could be rewritten as follows:

$$y_{it} = \beta_0 + \beta x_{it} + \alpha(s_{it} - \xi_{it}) + \theta_i + \varepsilon_{it}$$

the equivalent model at time (t+1) could be rewritten in a similar manner:

$$y_{it+1} = \beta_0 + \beta x_{it+1} + \alpha(s_{it+1} - \xi_{it+1}) + \theta_i + \varepsilon_{t+1}$$

the error terms ξ are unobserved and the above models cannot be estimated. Generally, we fit the following models to data:

$$y_{it} = \beta_0 + \beta x_{it} + \alpha s_{it} + \theta_i + (\varepsilon_{it} - \xi_{it}) \tag{10}$$

$$y_{it+1} = \beta_0 + \beta x_{it+1} + \alpha s_{it+1} + \theta_i + (\varepsilon_{t+1} - \xi_{it+1}) \tag{11}$$

equation (10) is the same as equation (9). However, by expressing the variance component model in this manner, it can be seen that the error term could be correlated with the explanatory variables included in equation (9). As discussed in Sub-section 3.7.2.2, such an association will lead to a serious specification problem which may lead to under-estimation of standard errors. If it were possible to operationalise this model, it would lead to explicit control for the time-variant omitted variables $\{\xi\}$. The values for $\{s'\}$ are not known, but the $\{s\}$ are observed and therefore are known. Rewrite equations (10) and (11) in the original form, as in equation (9):

$$y_{it} = \beta_0 + \beta x_{it} + \alpha s_{it} + \theta_i + \varepsilon_{it} \tag{12}$$

$$y_{it+1} = \beta_0 + \beta x_{it+1} + \alpha s_{it+1} + \theta_i + \varepsilon_{it+1} \tag{13}$$

This model can now be fitted and its parameters estimated using a combination of methods.

We condition on a sufficient statistic, e.g. for the continuous response variable by differencing equations (7) and (8) to eliminate θ (the conditional likelihood method, Sub-section 3.7.1.1). We use objective variables as instruments for the subjective variables in order to handle the explicit inclusion of the time-variant omitted variables and to resolve the specification problem.

Thus:

$$y_{it+1} - y_{it} = \beta(x_{it+1} - x_{it}) + \alpha(s_{it+1} - s_{it}) + (\varepsilon_{it+1} - \varepsilon_{it}) \tag{14}$$

As mentioned in Sub-section 3.7.2.3, only the error 'free' or objective measures, inside and outside the equation, can be used as instruments for the variables subject to error or for the subjective variables. There is nothing to prevent us from setting up utility functions, for each of the subjective variables in the model based, on time-invariant factors. For example, it is plausible that 'self-assessed health', 'self-assessed loneliness' or 'presence of friends in the

area' could be gender-related. The variable 'sex', which is an objective but a time-constant measure, could be used as one of the instruments to estimate these subjective variables, thereby utilising the information in the data set which was excluded from the analysis as a result of differencing.

APPENDIX X – SABRE COMMANDS

SABRE is a command driven program and recognises the following commands:

Syntax: ALPHA *number*
where *number* is a positive real number.
Purpose:
The ALPHA command sets the value of the orthogonality constant, which is used to trigger special action during the model fitting process.

***

Syntax: APPROXIMATE *number*
where *number* is a non-negative integer which is less than or equal to MAXITS.
Purpose:
The APPROXIMATE command sets the number of iterations which are to be performed using the Meilijson approximation to the Hessian matrix.

***

Syntax: ARITHMETIC *option*
where *option* is FAST or ACCURATE.
Purpose:
The ARITHMETIC command determines which method will be used in the calculation of the likelihood and its derivatives for mixture models.

***

Syntax: CASE *variable*
or

CASE *keyword=variable* [*keyword=variable*] where *keyword* is FIRST or SECOND.
Purpose:
The CASE command defines the variable which contains the case structure of the data. By default, this is taken to be the first name given in the list of variables specified in the DATA command; the CASE command is provided to override this default setting. The current case variable may be obtained by issuing the DISPLAY VARIABLES command.

***

Syntax: COMMENT *text*
Purpose:
The COMMENT command introduces the *text* as a comment into the SABRE run. This command is of most use when placed in INPUT files. Because SABRE looks for commands only on the first three spaces of the input line, comments can also be introduced by starting them on the fourth or higher space of a line.

***

Syntax: CONSTANT *variable*
or
CONSTANT *keyword=variable* [*keyword=variable* [*keyword=variable*]] where *keyword* is FIRST, SECOND or THIRD.
Purpose:
Specifies the names of the constants.

***

Syntax: CONVERGENCE *number*
where *number* is a positive real number.
Purpose:
The CONVERGENCE command sets the convergence criterion for subsequent model fitting using the FIT or LFIT command. If the difference in log-likelihood between subsequent iterations is less than *number*, then a convergence indicator is set.

***

Syntax: CORRELATED *option*
where *option* is NO or YES.
Purpose:
Specifies whether a correlated or uncorrelated model is to be fitted.

***

Syntax: CUTPOINTS *cut-point(s)*
where *cut-points* are a set of monotonically increasing real numbers.
The maximum number of cutpoints allowed is equal to the maximum number of parameters.
Purpose:
The CUTPOINTS command defines the starting values for the estimates of the cut-point parameters for the ordered response model.

***

Syntax: DATA *list of variables*
Purpose:
The DATA command has two purposes. Its primary purpose is to introduce a *list of variables* which are to be read by a subsequent READ command. The length of the variables is determined dynamically from the data introduced by the READ command. All variables are read as covariates; they can be subsequently converted to factors by the FACTOR command or transformed by the TRANSFORM command.

***

Syntax: DEFAULT
Purpose:
Sets all command arguments back to their default values.

***

Syntax: DELETE *list of variables*
Purpose:
This command is used to recover unwanted space. The variables specified in the *list of variables* will be deleted, and the space taken up by these variables will become available for other use.

***

Syntax: DEPEND *option*
where *option* is NO or YES.
Purpose:
Specifies a univariate random effects model with two scale parameters (SCALE1 and SCALE2). This command is used in conjunction with RVARIATE and two sets of interactions to specify separate equations dependent upon the value of a particular user-defined dummy variable. This dummy variable could be defined by: (i) the lagged response variable, (ii) a bivariate response variable indicator, or (iii) an initial response and non-initial response indicator.

***

Syntax: DER1 *option*
where *option* is NO or YES.
Purpose:
Specifies that subsequent random effects models should be fitted using only first derivatives of the log likelihood function.

***

Syntax: DISPLAY *option*
where *option* is ESTIMATES or LIMITS or MODEL or SETTINGS or VARIABLES.

Purpose:
The DISPLAY command provides information on the results of model fitting, the current settings, the current variables and other housekeeping information.

***

Syntax: ENDPOINTS *option* [*number1* [*number2*]]
where *option* is NO, LEFT, RIGHT or BOTH for binary models and NO or LEFT for Poisson models and *number1* and *number2* are optional non-negative real numbers.
Purpose:
The ENDPOINTS command determines which end-point parameters are to be included in the model. It applies only to univariate binary or univariate Poisson models.

***

Syntax: EQSCALE *option*
where *option* is NO or YES.
Purpose:
Specifies a bivariate random effects model in which both scale parameters are equal, so that the estimated random effects parameters in a subsequent model fit are SCALE (= SCALE1 = SCALE2) and CORR.

***

Syntax: FACTOR *variable factor* [*cutpoints(s)*]
where *cutpoints* are an optional set of real numbers.
Purpose:
The FACTOR command produces a set of dummy variables produced by considering the *variable* as a categorical variable. The set of dummy variables is referred to in SABRE by the name of the structure *factor*.

***

Syntax: FAMILY *option*
or
FAMILY *keyword=option* [*keyword=option* [*keyword=option*]] where *option* is B (for binomial), G (for Gaussian) or P (for Poisson) and *keyword* is FIRST, SECOND or THIRD.
Purpose:
FAMILY *option* specifies the distribution of the dependent variable in the univariate model.

***

Syntax: FEFIT *list of variables*
where *list of variables* is a set of time-varying covariates.

Purpose:
The FEFIT command fits a fixed effects model, taking as explanatory variables the list of variables specified as the argument to the command.

***

Syntax: FIT *list of variables*
where *list of variables* is a mixture of covariates, factors and pseudo factors.
Purpose:
The FIT command fits a random effects model (with optional end-points for univariate models).

***

Syntax: HISTOGRAM *variable* [*number*]
where *variable* is a covariate, factor or pseudo factor, and *number* is an optional integer between 2 and 11.
Purpose:
The HISTOGRAM command produces a rudimentary histogram of the *variable* into at most *number* groups. There may be less than *number* groups in the printed histogram due to the suppression of those groups with zero frequency.

***

Syntax: INITIAL *list of numbers*
Purpose:
The INITIAL command is used to specify the starting values for the explanatory variable parameters in a random effects model.

***

Syntax: INPUT *filename*
Purpose:
The INPUT command instructs SABRE to take input from the file specified in *filename* rather than from the previous input source. The file will in general consist of a sequence of SABRE commands; one on each line. On reaching the end of the input file, control will be returned to the terminal. It provides a convenient way of inputting the data and variable definitions into SABRE before returning control to the interactive session for subsequent model fitting.

***

Syntax: LFIT *list of variables*
where *list of variables* is a mixture of covariates, factors and pseudo factors.
Purpose:

The LFIT command fits a standard homogeneous model, taking as explanatory variables the list of variables specified as the argument to the command.

For ordered response models only, LFIT can be issued without arguments in order to fit a model with just cut-points and no covariates.

***

Syntax: LINK *option*
or
LINK *keyword=option* [*keyword=option* [*keyword=option*]] where *option* is L (for logit), P (for probit) or C (for complementary log-log). and *keyword* is FIRST, SECOND or THIRD.

Purpose:
LINK *option* specifies the link function for binomial models in the univariate case. (Gaussian and Poisson models have only a single (canonical) link function).

***

Syntax: LOOK *list of variables* [*number1 number2*]
where *list of variables* is a list of no more than six variables or factors, and *number1* and *number2* are optional positive integers with *number1* less than or equal to *number2*.

Purpose:
The LOOK command displays values of the listed variables in parallel. In the case of factors, the value displayed is the factor level. By default, all values of the variables are displayed. If *number1* and *number2* are specified, then only observations between *number1* and *number2* are printed.

***

Syntax: MASS *number*
or
MASS *keyword=number* [*keyword=number* [*keyword=number*]] where *number* is 1,2,4,6,8,10,12,14,16,20,24,28,32,36,40,44,48,56,64,72, 80,88,96,104,112,128,144,160,176,192,208,224,240 or 256 and *keyword* is FIRST, SECOND or THIRD.

Purpose:
MASS *number* sets the number of quadrature points used in the numerical integration as part of the model fitting process in univariate models instigated by the FIT command.

***

Syntax: MAXIMUM *number*
where *number* is a positive integer which is greater than or equal to APPROXIMATE.
Purpose:

The MAXIMUM command sets to *number* the maximum number of iterations which are to be performed by the model fitting algorithm.

***

Syntax: MODEL *option*
where *option* is UNIVARIATE, BIVARIATE or TRIVARIATE.
Purpose:
Specifies the type of model (univariate, bivariate or trivariate) to be fitted.

***

Syntax: NVAR *keyword=number* [*keyword=number*] where *number* is a positive integer and *keyword* is FIRST or SECOND.
Purpose:
NVAR FIRST=*number* specifies the number of variables in the first linear predictor for bivariate or trivariate models.

***

Syntax: OFFSET *variable*
where *variable* is the name of the offset variable.
Purpose:
The OFFSET command declares an a priori known component to be included in the linear predictor during model fitting. The offset itself is an explanatory variable - which may be both subject and time period specific - whose coefficient is fixed at 1.0, and is thus constant throughout the fitting process.

***

Syntax: ORDERED *option*
where *option* is NO or YES.
Purpose:
Specifies an ordered response model (if *option* is YES). This is an ordered probit if the LINK function is 'p' or an ordered logit if the LINK function is 'l'.

***

Syntax: OUTPUT [*filename*]
where *filename* is an optional argument defining the name of a file in which to write the output.
Purpose:
The OUTPUT command enables the writing of a log file containing a record of all screen output. This log file will contain all user commands and any screen displays resulting from the LOOK, HISTOGRAM, LFIT, FIT and DISPLAY commands.

***

Syntax: QUADRATURE *option*

where *option* is G or A.

Purpose:

Specifies the quadrature method to be used in subsequent random effects models, G for ordinary Gaussian quadrature or A for adaptive Gaussian quadrature.

***

Syntax: READ [*filename*]

where *filename* is an optional argument defining the name of a file in which the data is stored.

Purpose:

The READ command reads data values into the variables defined by a previous DATA command. The data values are read in free format, with numbers within a single row of the data matrix separated by spaces or newlines. Each new row of the data matrix needs to begin on a new line, but this is the only restriction.

***

Syntax: RESTART

Purpose:

Resets all parameter estimate starting values back to their default values.

***

Syntax: RHO *number*

or

RHO *keyword=number* [*keyword=number* [*keyword=number*]] where *number* is a positive real number and *keyword* is FIRST, SECOND or THIRD.

Purpose:

RHO *number* sets the initial value for the correlation parameter in bivariate models.

***

Syntax: RVARIATE *variable*

Purpose

Specifies the name of the response variate.

***

Syntax: SCALE *number*

or

SCALE *keyword=number* [*keyword=number* [*keyword=number*]] where *number* is a positive real number and *keyword* is FIRST, SECOND or THIRD.

Purpose:

SCALE *number* sets the initial value for the scale parameter in the univariate model to *number* for all subsequent models fitted by the FIT command.

***

Syntax: SIGMA *number*
or
SIGMA *keyword=number* [*keyword=number* [*keyword=number*]] where *number* is a positive real number and *keyword* is FIRST, SECOND or THIRD.
Purpose:
SIGMA *number* sets the initial value for the residual standard deviation in univariate linear (Gaussian) models.

***

Syntax: STOP
Purpose:
The SABRE run is terminated. The workspace is deleted, all files are closed and the screen is cleared. Control is returned to the operating system. In Windows, the SABRE window is shut down.

***

Syntax: TOLERANCE *number*
where *number* is a positive real number.
Purpose:
The TOLERANCE command sets to *number* the tolerance used in the matrix inversion routines to detect extrinsic aliasing and lack of positive semi-definiteness.

***

Syntax: TRACE [*filename*]
where *filename* is an optional argument defining the name of a file in which to write the trace output.
Purpose:
The TRACE command is analogous to the OUTPUT command and enables the writing of a trace file containing the values of the score/gradient vector of first derivatives of the log likelihood function at each iteration of the FIT.

***

Syntax:
TRANSFORM *variable function var1* or
TRANSFORM *variable var1 ^ number* or
TRANSFORM *variable var1 operator var2* or
TRANSFORM *variable var1 operator number*

where *variable* is the name of the transformed variable, *var1* and *var2* are explanatory variables, *number* is a real number, *function* is either *exp* or *log* and *operator* is either *, /, + or −.

Purpose:
The TRANSFORM command performs simple data transformations and also forms interactions between variables and/or factors.
***

Syntax: YVARIATE *variable*
Purpose:
The YVARIATE command defines the response variable which is to be used as the y-variate in subsequent model fitting. For binary models the y-variate must itself be binary (0,1), while for Poisson models it must be non-negative integer. There is no default to this command; it must be used before model fitting can commence. The current y-variate may be obtained by issuing the DISPLAY VARIABLES command.

BIOSKETCH

Said Shahtahmasebi, PhD, is currently Research Centre Director for the Good Life Research Centre Trust, Christchurch, and Research Leader, School of Health, WINTEC, Hamilton, New Zealand. He has held a number of research and consultancy posts within the university and health sector in the UK (National Health Service) and New Zealand. His work experiences cover a number of fields including public health, mental health, nursing, applied statistics and operational research, food and nutrition, gerontology, and disability. His area of interests and expertise are related to longitudinal modelling of health related behaviour. He has founded the Good Life Research Centre Trust to promote holistic research methodology to investigate health, social and behavioural issues relevant to the community. Email: said.shahtahmasebi@wintec.ac.nz.

Damon Berridge, PhD, is currently Senior Lecturer and Head of Applied Statistics Section, Lancaster University, Lancaster, UK. He has over twenty years of statistical research and consultancy in both academia and private sector.

INDEX

A

academic performance, 98
academics, 1
accidents, 1
accommodation, 39, 42, 79, 141, 142
accounting, 3, 41, 46, 98, 105, 114
accuracy, 78
adaptation, 143
adjustment, 2, 98
adolescence, 98, 129, 136, 137, 138
adolescents, 12, 116, 136
adulthood, 98, 137, 138
adults, 131
advertising, 107, 111
ageing, 43, 131, 134
agent, 114
aging, 131
alcohol, 3, 89, 97, 107, 109, 111, 114, 115, 137, 138
alcohol consumption, 97, 111, 114, 138
alcohol dependence, 138
alcohol use, 137, 138
algorithm, 77, 78, 167
alternative, 1, 22, 28, 42, 45, 51, 53, 71, 75, 81, 150
ambiguity, 22, 106
amphetamines, 111, 113
analytical framework, 12, 13, 97, 98
animal husbandry, 77
antidepressant, 129
anxiety, 14, 98, 106
argument, 126, 165, 166, 167, 168, 169
assessment, 39, 40, 45, 143
assumptions, xi, 134, 157
attitudes, 6, 43, 44, 99, 123, 135, 137, 155
Australia, 129
Austria, 132

authority, 75, 121
autism, 3
availability, 18, 33, 46, 50, 52, 54, 55, 69, 75, 77, 121, 143
awareness, 65, 72, 137

B

barbiturates, 113
beer, 3
behavior, vi, 129
beverages, 114
bias, 12, 35, 44, 45, 122, 126
blocks, 60
body shape, 122, 124, 125, 127
bowel, 3
brain, 3
breakfast, 113
breast cancer, 137
buffer, 54

C

campaigns, 114
cancer, 3
cannabis, 110, 111, 113, 114, 138
category a, 25, 37
causal relationship, 2, 36, 123
causality, 10, 23, 36, 44, 45, 98
cell, 15, 18, 28
Census, 133
childrearing, 143
children, 14, 15, 16, 19, 23, 24, 28, 38, 78, 135, 136, 141, 142, 143
chronic illness, 133
cigarette smoking, 135, 136, 137

classification, 15, 16, 18, 73, 110
classroom, 123
classrooms, 123
clinical trials, 1
close relationships, 143
cluster analysis, 45
clustering, 123, 126
clusters, 57, 123
cognitive impairment, 132
cohort, 132, 136, 138
coke, 113
community, 12, 13, 16, 17, 23, 24, 25, 26, 27, 28, 29, 30, 31, 32, 33, 34, 35, 40, 41, 44, 46, 81, 130, 141, 142, 143, 144, 146, 171
comorbidity, 136
competence, 54, 75
competition, 54, 61
complex interactions, 43, 121
complexity, 13, 72, 75, 121
components, 68, 81, 134
composition, 16, 19, 24, 28, 38, 47, 55, 61, 66, 67, 70, 141, 142
computer software, 77
computing, 1, 77, 80, 130
concentrates, 26, 79
conditioning, 58, 59, 69, 70, 75
confidence, 98, 104, 105, 106, 122, 123, 124, 126
confidence interval, 104, 105, 122
confusion, xi, 10
Congress, vi
consciousness, 123
construction, 44
consumption, 111, 137
contingency, 15
control, xii, 5, 11, 13, 17, 18, 23, 24, 33, 37, 38, 40, 43, 45, 48, 53, 54, 56, 58, 59, 66, 67, 69, 72, 73, 75, 77, 80, 98, 101, 106, 110, 121, 122, 129, 158, 165
convergence, 83, 162
convergence criteria, 83
correlation, 22, 57, 91, 98, 106, 118, 152, 168
correlations, 67
cost-benefit analysis, 135
covering, 45, 134
crack, 113
critical thinking, xi
criticism, 10, 21
cross-sectional study, 126
culture, xi, 114, 115, 119
cumulative distribution function, 149

D

daily living, 46, 52, 61, 66, 67, 70, 142
data analysis, vi, 107
data collection, 4, 126
data set, 18, 23, 45, 46, 47, 49, 52, 57, 60, 64, 81, 101, 107, 109, 142, 159
data structure, 57, 84, 91
database, 12, 15
death, 13, 14, 22, 23, 25, 27, 29, 31, 33, 34, 35, 36, 37, 38, 39, 41, 42, 121, 127, 145, 147
death rate, 14, 25, 37, 39
deaths, 36
decomposition, 30
definition, 28, 126
dementia, 44, 132
density, 36, 149, 151
dependent variable, 164
depression, 4, 14, 44, 132
derivatives, 161, 163, 169
diffusion, 116
dimensionality, 45
disability, xi, 2, 3, 4, 82, 171
discrete data, 79, 134
distribution, 22, 36, 46, 80, 81, 83, 91, 101, 111, 146, 149, 153, 157, 164
diversity, 117, 118, 119
divorce, 141, 142
double counting, 123
drinking pattern, 12, 107, 112, 114, 138
drug use, 107, 138
drugs, 99, 107, 111, 112, 137
duration, 7, 13, 33, 34, 35, 36, 39, 41, 42, 45, 47, 64, 79, 105, 114, 134, 149

E

earnings, 129
economic activity, 77
economic resources, 46, 52, 56, 142
economic status, 14
economics, 84
ecstasy, 111, 113, 114
Education, 136, 137
educational attainment, 78
elderly, 2, 5, 6, 7, 8, 12, 14, 23, 24, 25, 26, 28, 29, 31, 34, 39, 42, 43, 44, 45, 49, 54, 57, 60, 63, 68, 116, 126, 130, 131, 132, 138, 139, 143, 149
elderly population, 132

employment, 2, 130, 135
employment status, 2
encouragement, xii, 114
England, 99, 131, 133, 135
English Language, xii
environment, xi, 135, 136
environmental factors, 122, 125
environmental tobacco, 137
epilepsy, 134
estimating, 70, 134, 136
estimation process, 78, 156
ethnic groups, 116, 119
ethnicity, 12, 21, 23, 33, 40, 41, 50, 51, 91, 92, 116, 117, 118, 119, 138
evidence-based policy, 1
exclusion, 35, 58
exercise, 59, 65, 121, 146, 156
expertise, 171
exposure, 105, 111, 117, 118, 127

F

factor analysis, 45
failure, 22, 80, 145, 149
family, xi, 2, 16, 24, 26, 28, 38, 42, 47, 50, 55, 61, 66, 67, 70, 81, 98, 100, 101, 102, 103, 104, 105, 106, 110, 111, 112, 122, 123, 124, 125, 127, 136, 138, 141, 142, 143
family environment, 98
family life, 111
family members, 104, 127
family relationships, 143
feedback, xi, 7, 80, 97, 98, 127
feelings, 98, 106, 143
females, 15, 23, 29, 107, 111
flexibility, 44, 45, 72, 80, 97, 101
food, 100, 101, 102, 103, 104, 105, 113, 122, 123, 124, 127, 171
freedom, 49, 93, 94, 95, 111
friendship, 7, 45, 116, 118, 119, 123, 130
frustration, xi
fulfillment, 44
funding, 12

G

gender, 14, 37, 38, 91, 99, 100, 104, 108, 122, 159
gene, 83, 84
gerontology, 171

governance, xi
government, 111
grouping, 121, 126, 136
groups, 14, 23, 33, 36, 79, 111, 122, 165
growth, 3
guidance, 123
guidelines, 114

H

happiness, 44, 132
hazards, 150
health care, 5, 7
health effects, 16
health ratings, 66
health status, 1, 23, 33, 42
heart disease, 106, 114
heavy drinking, 108, 111
heroin, 113
heterogeneity, 6, 9, 44, 45, 56, 58, 59, 67, 69, 72, 73, 75, 77, 83, 97, 98, 101, 104, 105, 106, 107, 114, 115, 117, 134, 135, 153, 157
high school, 137
histogram, 83, 165
House, 28
household composition, 14, 15, 21, 50
households, 143
housing, 14
hypothesis, 1, 11, 23, 45, 117
hypothesis test, 1, 11, 23, 45

I

identification, 21, 135
immigrants, 116, 138
implementation, 1, 136
incidence, 2, 123, 132, 136
inclusion, 21, 22, 28, 32, 36, 39, 43, 46, 48, 53, 61, 62, 65, 66, 69, 70, 75, 121, 122, 143, 158
income, xi, 2, 14, 15, 21, 39, 41, 44, 50, 51, 84, 127, 138, 142
independence, 27, 60, 65, 75, 92, 98, 117, 118
independent variable, 109
indication, 29, 51, 122
indicators, 14, 126
indices, 21
individual character, 45, 48, 106, 107
individual characteristics, 45, 48, 106, 107
industry, 1, 115, 129

inertia, 80
infertility, 77
initiation, 106, 137, 138
innovation, xii, 119
insight, xi, 35, 41, 48, 72, 98, 122, 127
instruments, 69, 70, 71, 75, 155, 158
integration, 14, 152, 166
intelligence, 14
intentions, 135, 136
interaction, 7, 14, 23, 45, 92
interaction effect, 23
interaction effects, 23
interactions, 14, 29, 43, 99, 109, 115, 123, 163, 170
interval, 59, 122, 149
intervention, 44
interview, 2, 34, 45, 121, 122, 141
intuition, 63
inversion, 169
ionizing radiation, 137
isolation, 1, 14, 15, 16, 46, 143
iteration, 50, 169

J

justification, 52, 111

L

labour, 79, 84, 157
labour market, 79
language, xi, 119
legislation, 111
life satisfaction, 14
lifestyle, 111, 143
limitation, 9, 46, 49, 60, 99, 129
linear model, 10, 46, 79, 80, 81, 91
linear modeling, 10
links, 95, 106
listening, 12, 116
local government, 43
location, 91, 92, 116, 118, 119
loneliness, 2, 6, 7, 14, 15, 16, 17, 31, 33, 38, 45, 132, 141, 142, 143, 157, 158
longevity, 2, 14, 21, 37
longitudinal study, 11, 49, 107, 131, 132

M

Mackintosh, 137

males, 15, 29, 107, 111
marijuana, 137, 138
marital status, 15, 21, 46, 52, 55, 142
marketing, 137
marriage, 79
masking, 107
mathematics, xi, 1
matrix, 27, 37, 156, 161, 168, 169
matrix algebra, 37
measurement, 14, 64, 69, 75, 126, 135, 155, 157
measurement bias, 69
measures, 6, 10, 15, 26, 38, 40, 43, 44, 45, 46, 47, 50, 51, 52, 53, 54, 55, 56, 60, 61, 62, 63, 64, 66, 67, 69, 70, 71, 72, 84, 98, 115, 137, 142, 158
measures of perception, 137
media, 3, 106, 114, 127
membership, 77, 78
memory, 3
men, 6, 14, 30, 37
mental disorder, 132
mental health, 45, 52, 54, 56, 66, 142, 171
mental illness, 4
mental state, 132
messages, 138
middle class, 23, 141, 142
migrants, 23, 32
migration, 77, 79
mixing, 101, 111, 153, 157
mobile phone, 119
mobility, 14, 44, 116, 134, 136
modeling, 13, 35, 49, 136
money, 100, 101, 102, 103, 104, 105, 106, 109, 110, 112, 122, 123, 124, 125
morale, 2, 5, 6, 10, 11, 14, 15, 16, 17, 44, 45, 46, 47, 48, 49, 50, 51, 52, 53, 54, 55, 56, 57, 58, 60, 61, 62, 63, 64, 65, 68, 69, 71, 72, 73, 74, 75, 121, 132, 143, 157
morbidity, 14, 33, 40, 106
mortality, 14, 33, 37, 39, 40, 106, 131, 149
mortality rate, 14, 33, 37, 149
motivation, xii
movement, 33

N

National Health Service, 99, 171
nerve, 3
Netherlands, 129, 135
network, 14, 15, 16, 17, 24, 28, 33, 37, 38, 46, 50, 51, 92, 116, 117, 118, 119, 141, 143, 144

networking, 119
New Zealand, 3, 114, 129, 171
noise, 44
non-smokers, 84, 99, 108, 126
nursing, 171
nutrition, 99, 171

O

objectivity, 115
observations, 8, 9, 11, 15, 33, 43, 46, 52, 64, 72, 93, 99, 105, 109, 114, 116, 129, 152, 166
old age, 5, 10, 11, 13, 14, 15, 16, 17, 21, 22, 25, 26, 31, 33, 39, 43, 44, 45, 49, 54, 55, 58, 60, 63, 69, 71, 72, 75, 121, 129, 130, 132, 133, 139, 143, 149
older people, 132
operating system, 169
operator, 169, 170
optimization, 37
ordinal data, 131
orthogonality, 161

P

pain, 44, 132, 133
parameter, 22, 25, 27, 29, 31, 32, 33, 37, 38, 50, 51, 53, 54, 58, 61, 62, 69, 73, 75, 80, 83, 101, 103, 104, 105, 111, 114, 117, 118, 122, 123, 145, 152, 168, 169
parameter estimates, 22, 25, 29, 31, 32, 33, 37, 38, 50, 51, 53, 54, 61, 62, 75, 83, 103, 105, 111, 117, 122, 123
parameter estimation, 27, 80
parental influence, 106, 123, 137
parental involvement, 111
parental smoking, 98, 115, 135, 137
parents, 112, 114, 122, 124, 125, 126
pathways, 105, 114
peer group, 123
perceptions, 6, 43, 75, 135, 138, 155
personality, 2, 43, 44, 98, 115, 126
physical exercise, 99
physical health, 34, 43, 46, 52, 56, 63, 66, 67, 68, 73, 142
pilot study, 133
policy makers, xi, 115
policy making, xii
politics, 127

poor, 1, 6, 14, 17, 22, 23, 25, 29, 31, 32, 34, 37, 39, 41, 44, 50, 52, 62, 63, 74, 77, 141, 142, 145, 146
population, xii, 8, 13, 79, 106, 118, 133, 134
positive relation, 84
positive relationship, 84
poverty, 2
power, 21, 42, 50, 51, 115
prediction, 138
predictors, 136, 137
pregnancy, 136
prejudice, 34, 80
pressure, 105, 107, 111, 115, 123
prestige, 4
prevention, 114, 136, 137
private sector, 171
probability, 2, 7, 10, 11, 18, 22, 25, 26, 27, 29, 30, 31, 32, 35, 36, 45, 98, 101, 104, 130, 145, 146, 149, 151, 152, 153
probability density function, 149, 152, 153
probability distribution, 10, 30, 31, 32, 36, 149
production, 135
prognosis, 44
program, 36, 37, 78, 81, 131, 134, 139, 161
prosperity, 116
protective factors, 137
psychological variables, 98, 122, 143
psychological well-being, 98, 136
public health, 171
public policy, 134
pupil, 123

Q

quality of life, 13, 33, 37, 40, 44, 45, 54, 71, 126, 133

R

race, 138
random errors, 155
range, 44, 45, 99, 115, 116
rating scale, 54, 61, 66, 67, 70, 142
ratings, 142
real numbers, 162, 164
recall, 121
recognition, 132
recurrence, 132
refining, 121

regression, 10, 24, 25, 26, 34, 49, 50, 57, 58, 65, 71, 80, 83, 98, 100, 104, 105, 109, 115, 122, 124, 133, 135, 136, 137, 145, 155, 156
relationship, 2, 7, 10, 13, 15, 16, 17, 21, 23, 24, 33, 37, 38, 44, 48, 50, 56, 72, 98, 105, 107, 115, 127, 138, 143
relationships, 2, 5, 15, 17, 21, 23, 24, 37, 43, 44, 45, 48, 49, 53, 64, 65, 73, 75, 98, 105, 115, 143, 149
relatives, 14, 31, 39, 47, 50, 55, 61, 62, 63, 66, 67, 70, 71, 72, 74, 75, 141, 142, 143
religion, 138
rent, 17, 52
reputation, 138
residuals, 10
resilience, 98, 106, 137
resources, 35, 61, 66, 67, 70
restaurants, 111
retirement, 13, 16, 23, 32, 141, 142
revenue, 111
risk, 3, 39, 56, 79, 80, 98, 106, 122, 123, 131, 135, 137, 138
risk assessment, 98
risk factors, 138
risk-taking, 98, 135
routines, 14, 169
Royal Society, 1
R-squared, 47, 52, 55, 56, 61, 62, 63, 71, 72
rural areas, 14, 34

S

sample, 10, 12, 15, 22, 25, 29, 35, 37, 44, 46, 49, 52, 53, 78, 80, 89, 91, 92, 99, 101, 104, 105, 107, 110, 111, 116, 137, 145, 152
sampling, 9, 10, 77, 123, 138
satisfaction, 43, 44
school, 78, 98, 99, 112, 122, 123, 135, 136, 137
school activities, 99
school adjustment, 136
scores, 49, 52, 54, 56, 60, 63, 141
search, 1, 13
secondary data, 97
secondary schools, 99
selecting, 11, 22, 45
self-assessment, 42, 55
self-esteem, 46, 98, 106, 115, 122, 123, 135
self-image, 46
senile dementia, 132
series, 22, 36, 44, 121, 134
shape, 122, 127

sibling, 16, 143
siblings, 141, 142
SIGMA, 169
significance level, 21, 53, 103, 104, 111
signs, 41
similarity, 126
smoke, 89, 97, 98, 101, 104, 112, 123, 127, 137
smokers, 84, 98, 99, 103, 106, 108, 123, 126
smoking, 2, 12, 44, 83, 84, 97, 98, 99, 100, 101, 104, 105, 106, 107, 108, 110, 111, 115, 121, 122, 123, 124, 125, 126, 130, 135, 136, 137, 138
smoothing, 18
social attitudes, 115
social behaviour, 7, 115
social class, 5, 14, 15, 33, 37, 39, 41, 51, 122, 142
social group, 98, 123
social influence, 122
social network, 34
social participation, 46
social policy, 116
social resources, 46, 52
social sciences, 5
social status, 122
social support, 44, 45, 46
software, 21, 27, 70, 77, 78, 146, 151
solvents, 113
spectrum, 14
speech, 12, 116
stability, 138
stages, 38, 70, 111
standard deviation, 111, 169
standard error, 33, 37, 57, 83, 103, 105, 111, 117, 123, 124, 158
statistical inference, 10
statistics, xi, 1, 10, 65, 171
stimulus, 92, 93, 117, 118
strength, 27
stress, 106, 137
subjectivity, 115
substance abuse, 137
substance use, 137, 138
substitution, 37, 53, 110
subtraction, 59
suicide, 4, 129
suicide attempts, 129
suicide rate, 4
suppression, 165
survival, 7, 11, 13, 14, 15, 16, 17, 18, 21, 22, 24, 25, 26, 27, 29, 30, 31, 32, 33, 34, 35, 36, 37, 38, 39,

40, 41, 42, 43, 121, 126, 130, 131, 136, 142, 143, 146, 149, 150
survival rate, 15, 23, 42, 142
survivors, 12, 15, 25, 41, 45, 60, 121, 130, 131
systems, 14

T

technology, 119
telephone, 141, 142, 143
tenants, 14, 142
tenure, 8, 14, 15, 17, 19, 24, 28, 38, 39, 40, 41, 42, 47, 50, 51, 52, 55, 61, 66, 67, 70, 141, 142
test statistic, 15, 21, 22, 23, 28, 37, 38, 49, 50, 53, 55, 59, 61, 65, 70, 109, 110
text messaging, 119
threshold, 27
time periods, 134
time series, 80, 121
tobacco, 111, 135, 137, 138
trade, 77, 78
trade union, 77, 78
training, 78
traits, 2
transformation, 18, 46, 145
transformations, 21, 170
transition, 136, 137
translation, 2
transport, 141, 142, 143
trial, 136

U

unemployment, 10, 78, 79, 80, 112, 130, 135
unemployment rate, 79
United States, 137
US Department of Health and Human Services, 137

V

vaccine, 3
values, 5, 10, 15, 17, 18, 22, 27, 29, 33, 38, 39, 45, 47, 49, 50, 52, 53, 55, 59, 60, 61, 62, 63, 70, 71, 74, 83, 84, 90, 103, 109, 111, 138, 155, 156, 157, 158, 162, 163, 165, 166, 168, 169
variability, 98
variable factor, 164
variance, 45, 57, 69, 157, 158
variation, 5, 7, 8, 10, 11, 12, 13, 22, 42, 44, 50, 53, 54, 58, 60, 72, 73, 77, 90, 101, 106, 111, 115, 116, 117, 118, 150
vector, 10, 57, 58, 152, 169
village, 125
vocabulary, xi
voluntary organizations, 143
voting, 77

W

wages, 78
Wales, 12, 45, 130, 133, 134, 138, 139, 142
Wallace and Silver (1988), 5
weakness, 1
web, 78
winning, 2
women, 14, 30, 37, 130
worry, 17, 101, 104, 105, 106, 109, 122, 123, 127, 141
writing, 21, 167, 169

Y

young adults, 99